Recent Advances in

Paediatrics

22

Edited by

Timothy J. David MB ChB MD PhD FRCP FRCPCH DCH

Professor of Child Health and Paediatrics,
University of Manchester;
Honorary Consultant Paediatrician,
Booth Hall Children's Hospital, Manchester, UK

© 2005 Royal Society of Medicine Press Ltd

Published by the Royal Society of Medicine Press Ltd
1 Wimpole Street, London W1G 0AE, UK
Tel: +44 (0) 20 7290 2921; Fax: +44 (0) 20 7290 2929
E-mail: publishing@rsm.ac.uk
Website: www.rsmpress.co.uk

British Library Cataloguing in Publication Data
A catalogue record for this book is available from the British Library

ISBN 1–85315–597-7

ISSN 0-309-0140

Distribution in Europe and Rest of World:
Marston Book Services Ltd, PO Box 269, Abingdon, Oxon OX14 4YN, UK
Tel: +44 (0) 1235 465500; Fax: +44 (0) 1235 465555
E-mail: direct.order@marston.co.uk

Distribution in the USA and Canada:
Royal Society of Medicine Press Ltd, c/o Jamco Distribution Inc
1401 Lakeway Drive, Lewisville, TX 75057, USA
Tel: +1 800 538 1287; Fax: +1 972 353 1303
E-mail: jamco@majors.com

Distribution in Australia and New Zealand:
Elsevier Australia
30-52 Smidmore Street, Marrickville NSW 2204, Australia
Tel: +61 2 9517 8999; Fax: +61 2 9517 2249
E-mail: service@elsevier.com.au

Commissioning editor: Peter Richardson
Editorial assistant: Shirley Mukisa
Production by GM & BA Haddock, Midlothian, UK

Printed in Great Britain by Bell & Bain, Glasgow, UK

Contents

Contents

Preface

The aim of *Recent Advances in Paediatrics* is to provide a review of important topics and help doctors keep abreast of developments in the subject. The book is intended for the practising clinician, those in specialty training, and doctors preparing for specialty examinations. The book is sold very widely in Britain, Europe, North America and Asia, and the contents and authorship are selected with this very broad readership in mind. There are 15 chapters which cover a variety of general paediatric, neonatal and community paediatric areas. As usual, the selection of topics has veered towards those of general rather than special interest.

The final chapter, an annotated literature review, is a personal selection of key articles and useful reviews published in 2003. Comment about a paper is sometimes as important as the original article, so when a paper has been followed by interesting or important correspondence, or accompanied by a useful editorial, this is also referred to. As with the choice of subjects for the main chapters, the selection of articles has inclined towards those of general rather than special interest. There is, however, special emphasis on community paediatrics and medicine in the tropics, as these two important areas tend to be less well covered in general paediatric journals. Trying to reduce to an acceptable size the short-list of particularly interesting articles is an especially difficult task. Each topic in the literature review section is asterisked in the index, so selected publications on (for example) child abuse can be identified easily, as can any parts of the book that touch on the topic.

I am indebted to the authors for their hard work, prompt delivery of manuscripts and patience in dealing with my queries and requests. I would also like to thank my secretaries Angela Smithies and Valerie Smith, and Gill Haddock of the RSM Press, for all their help. Working on a book such as this makes huge inroads into one's spare time, and my special thanks go to my wife and sons for all their support.

Professor Timothy J. David
University Department of Child Health,
Booth Hall Children's Hospital, Manchester M9 7AA, UK
E-mail: t.david@netcomuk.co.uk

2004

1

1

Abusive head trauma

Abusive head trauma in infants and small children is the most common fatal manifestation of child abuse. Many areas of controversy exist in the diagnosis of abusive head trauma. This monograph will review the epidemiology of abusive head trauma, some basic biomechanical properties of brain tissue, the diagnosis of abusive head trauma, and the outcomes of children who were victims of abusive head trauma. Management of head trauma will not be discussed.

INCIDENCE

Barlow and Minns conducted a prospective cohort study of non-accidental head injury for one year in Wales.[1] They found it to be 24.6 cases per 100,000 population, with a 95% confidence interval (95% CI) of 14.9–38.5. There were 19 cases in their population, with a median age of 2.2 months. No children over 1 year-of-age died of abusive head trauma.

Another incidence study was published by Jayawant and colleagues in 1998.[2] This study was a retrospective case series of inflicted subdural haematomas in children under 2 years-of-age. they found an incidence of 10.1 subdural haematomas per 100,000 population (95% CI, 5.3–19.2). In children younger than 1 year, the incidence was 21 per 100,000. Male children were shown to be at increased risk. Children age 2.2–8.7 months were also at increased risk.

A prospective, population-based study was done in the State of North Carolina in the US.[3] Of the serious or fatal traumatic brain injuries in children under 2 years-of-age, 53% were found to be non-accidental, inflicted injuries.

Carole Jenny MD MBA
Professor of Pediatrics, Brown Medical School, Hasbro Children's Hospital, 593 Eddy Street, Providence, RI 02903, USA
E-mail: cjenny@lifespan.org

The incidence of inflicted brain injuries in the first two years of life was 17.0 (95% CI, 133–20.7) per 100,000 person-years. Infants less than 1 year-of age had an incidence of 29.7 (95% CI, 22.9-36.7) per 100,000 person-years.

Children with abusive head trauma were more likely to be male, of a minority race, and born to mothers less than 21 years-of-age. In another study from North Carolina, the incidence of abusive head trauma was shown to increase after a natural disaster.[4]

The results of these studies are surprisingly concordant given the very diverse areas covered and methods used.

BIOMECHANICS OF HEAD AND BRAIN INJURIES

Brain tissue is non-compressible but highly deformable.[5] Tension and compression of brain tissue lead to focal injuries, and wide-spread injury results from rotational forces. Holbourn et al.[5] determined that patterns of brain injury also depend on the duration of the injurious event. Short-duration events lead to focal injuries, while long duration events can cause deeper injury in the brain.

When children present with abusive head trauma, caregivers often falsely describe the injuries as resulting from a short fall. However, children have to be shown to be able to survive much longer falls than adults, and to be less likely to sustain serious injury at falls from any height.[6] One study found that 'death' was not the outcome in children unless the fall exceeded 30.5 m (100 ft) in height.

Foust et al.[7] studied 110 free-falls of children: 26 were 'head-first' falls and 82% of the falling children impacted rigid surfaces. In small children, they predicted that 11.4 kg (25 lb) times 30.5 m (100 ft) was the limit to exceed for death from free-falls. In general, the likelihood of a child sustaining a serious head injury from a short household fall is slight.

The amount of rotational ('whiplash') acceleration required to cause brain injury in the absence of impact has been studied in animal models.[8–12] However, similar data do not exist for immature primates. The brain of the human infant has a higher water content and lower protein content than that of the adult. The young infant's neck is incapable of supporting or protecting the head. No comparable animal model exists.

Gennarelli and co-workers recognised patterns of loading that were more likely to result in subdural haematomas[11] or more likely to cause diffuse axonal injury.[13] Coronal rotation and long-duration events were more likely to cause diffuse axonal injury. Saggital rotation was more likely to cause subdural haematomas.

Overall, the literature supports the following facts:[14]

1. Primary brain injury can result from mechanical forces.

2. Contact forces lead to focal brain injuries.

3. Translational inertial injuries cause focal brain injuries.

4. Rotational inertial injuries cause diffuse brain injuries such as loss of consciousness, concussion, or diffuse axonal injury.

5. Translational and inertial brain injuries include coup–contracoup injuries, cerebral lacerations, intracerebral haemorrhages, subdural haematomas, subarachnoid haemorrhages, and diffuse petechial haemorrhages of brain tissue.

6. Primary head injuries include soft tissue injuries, subgaleal haemorrhages, skull fractures, epidural haematomas, subdural haematomas, subarachonoid haemorrhages, diffuse axonal injury, cortical contusions, and lacerations or tears of brain tissue.

7. Secondary brain injury is not the direct result of mechanical forces. Secondary brain injuries include hypoxic–ischaemic injuries, secondary metabolic changes, and cerebral oedema.

CLINICAL PRESENTATION

Various clusters of signs and symptoms have been considered more predictive of abusive head trauma, including some or all of the following:

- Subdural haematoma

- Grey–white matter shearing tears of brain tissue

- Diffuse traumatic axonal injury

- Retinal haemorrhages, particularly when found throughout the area of the retina and involving many layers of retina

- Traumatic axonal pathology at the cervicomedullary junction

- Optic nerve sheath haemorrhage

- Apnoea

- Skull fractures or other evidence of impact to the head.

A recent North American panel convened by the National Institutes of Health proposed the following classification of types of abusive head trauma summarised in Box 1.[15]

Some experts contend that shaking alone does not injure infants' brains, but impact is required to generate the necessary forces.[16,17] These studies are based on anthropomorphic testing devices (crash test dummies). The lack of biofidelity of the model might cause the results to be questioned.[18] In addition, the authors consider only the effect of a single shake as opposed to the strains in brain tissue that accumulate over time with the repeated events occurring during an episode of shaking. A wealth of clinical data confirms that shaking has been identified as one of the mechanisms of that can lead to brain injury in abused infants.[19–23]

These factors – the increased vulnerability of the infant brain, the effect of repetitive cyclic impulses, and the prolonged time of application of force in shaking – are likely to increase the occurrence of injury in shaking episodes with or without impact.

Since using the term 'shaken baby syndrome' implies a known mechanism of trauma, using the more general term 'abusive head trauma' may be

---

Box 1 The National Institutes of Health's classification of types of abusive head trauma[15]

Shaking injury or shaken baby syndrome

Traumatic brain injury

No evidence of impact on clinical or radiographic examination

May have rib fractures, metaphyseal chip fractures of the long bones, retinal haemorrhages, and/or fingertip bruising

No other obvious major injuries

Unwitnessed trauma with no consistent history for injury, social work or judicial determination of abuse, or confession of abuse

Shaking-impact syndrome

Includes all of the above, except must have evidence of impact which may include skull fractures or scalp injuries seen clinically, forensically or radiographically

Battered child with inflicted brain injury

Traumatic brain injury with or without impact

Obvious clinical signs of past or current inflicted non-brain injuries, including injuries to other major organ systems

Unwitnessed trauma with no consistent history for the injury, social work or judicial determination of abuse, or confession of abuse

---

warranted. This term refers to major head trauma that occurs in the absence of a reasonable history of accidental injury, and does not infer the specific mechanism of injury. However, it remains important to warn parents about the potential of shaking to cause brain injury as part of the child abuse prevention information they receive.

Proposed non-abusive mechanisms for the above cluster of signs and symptoms in the absence of a viable history of significant injury have been proposed. These include including isolated hypoxia and short falls. Each of these hypothesised mechanisms will be considered separately.

HYPOXIA

Geddes has hypothesised that hypoxia alone can cause subdural 'leakage' through damaged dural vessels.[24] Other components of the cluster of symptoms noted above have not been studied. In particular, she did not look for the presence of retinal haemorrhages in her reported cases. This hypothesis is very controversial and not generally accepted. Geddes reached her conclusions by studying aborted fetuses and infants who died of complex medical illnesses such as Gram-negative sepsis. To extrapolate these findings to normal healthy children is not likely to yield valid conclusions.[25] Also, many conditions associated with anoxia such as prematurity and drowning are not known to be associated with subdural haematomas.

SHORT FALLS

It has been hypothesised that short, simple childhood falls can be the cause of the cluster of symptoms described above. Cases have been reported where children have died from witnessed short falls. In one reported series, only one of 18 cases of death from short falls did not have complicating factors such as bleeding disorders or rotational acceleration as part of the event.[26]

Several factors suggest that death from a short fall is an exceedingly uncommon event.[27–29] In fact, there is a large body of data showing that witnessed short falls are usually innocuous. Physical findings in witnessed short falls have not been shown to be the same as findings in inflicted trauma such as extensive retinal haemorrhages. Prospective studies show that extensive retinal haemorrhages do not occur in minor accidental injuries,[30] and are even uncommon in cases of severe, complicated injuries such as those occurring in major automobile accidents.[31,32]

RETINAL HAEMORRHAGES

Retinal haemorrhages can be categorised by the amount of blood present, the level of retinal layers involved, and the distribution of the haemorrhages.[33] Retinal haemorrhages in abusive head trauma are more likely to be subretinal, intraretinal, and preretinal, and are more likely to be found distributed throughout the retina out to the ora serrata. Wide-spread retinal haemorrhages in infants are more likely due to inflicted trauma. Examination by an ophthalmologist is essential if abuse is suspected.

No particular protocol exists for accurately dating retinal haemorrhages. Rate of healing varies depending on the size of the bleed, the layers of the retina involved, and the mechanism of causation of the haemorrhage.

Traumatic retinoschisis is another phenomenon observed in abusive head trauma, particularly in infants who have been shaken. It was first reported by Greenwald and colleagues in 1986.[30] These are cystic lesions with haemorrhagic edges. They may be related to stretching of the nerve fibre during acceleration/deceleration events. Traumatic retinoschisis has never been reported to occur in any setting other than abusive head trauma and severe crush injuries.

In abusive head trauma, 85% of children have retinal haemorrhages – 61% are intraretinal, preretinal and/or subretinal and 32% have retinoschisis. Papiloedema only occurs in 8% of cases. Often retinal haemorrhages are asymmetrical, and occasionally unilateral.[34]

The biomechanics of retinal haemorrhages in abusive head trauma is debated. The most reasonable hypothesis is that the acceleration and deceleration of the orbit puts traction on the retina, which is tightly attached to the vitreous in infants. Vasoregulatory dysfunction and shearing of retinal vessels may be involved.

OUTCOME

Several studies have looked at long-term clinical and functional effects of abusive head trauma. Ewing-Cobbs et al.[35] compared the outcomes of inflicted and non-inflicted neurotrauma in children. Abuse compared to accidental injury accounted for 90% of the variance in cognition. In children less than 1 year-of-age, abuse was the most powerful predictor of decreased cognitive function.

Barlow and colleagues studied 25 survivors of abusive head trauma – 68% had significant morbidity and 36% were severely disabled requiring long-term care. Disabilities included speech and language problems, cognitive deficits, motor deficits, epilepsy, and visual deficits. Of the children re-examined at a later date, all exhibited more serious deficits as they aged.

Other studies support the fact that children suffering abusive head trauma have a worse outcome overall than children suffering non-intentional head trauma.[36,37]

TIMING OF INFANT HEAD INJURY RELATED TO ONSET OF SYMPTOMS

Generally, it is agreed that young victims of moderate-to-severe head trauma become rapidly, clearly and persistently ill. Willman et al.[38] studied Glasgow Coma Scores in infants and young children sustaining serious head injuries in automobile accidents. They confirmed the immediate and progressive development of symptoms after serious head injury. The severity of the presenting symptoms is most likely proportional to the severity of the injury, with the exception of symptoms caused by epidural haematomas. Initial lucid intervals are common in epidural haematomas.

On the other hand, timing of onset of symptoms after inflicted trauma can be variable and inconsistent, particularly in less severe incidents. Patients who 'talk and die' are more likely to have focal brain injuries rather than diffuse injuries.[39] Expanding mass lesions or resultant hypoxia can delay onset of severe symptoms. However, after serious abusive head trauma, most children will show some level of symptoms immediately.

Some waxing and waning of symptoms may occur after serious injury. Non-specific symptoms are hard to assess, particularly in young infants. A recent study examined the onset of symptoms in cases of infant head trauma where the perpetrator confessed abusing the child. In 91% of the cases, the infant became symptomatic immediately after being abused.[40]

DIAGNOSIS

Symptoms of abusive head trauma occur on a spectrum from very mild to immediately fatal, depending on the nature of the injury and the vulnerability of the victim. The person presenting the child for care usually either does not know the child has been injured, or, if he or she does know, does not provide an accurate history. If the child presents with a history of head trauma, the history is usually given that the child suffered a minor insult, such as rolling off a couch or falling from standing. The assessment of the severity of the injury expected after such an event to the seriousness of the presenting signs and symptoms then leads the examiner to suspect abusive head trauma.

One study has pointed out the difficulty in making the diagnosis of abusive head trauma.[41] That study looked at previous missed abusive head trauma that had occurred in 173 cases where abusive head trauma was diagnosed. Of the abused children, 31% had previously suffered abusive head trauma and had been seen by a physician who missed the diagnosis. Risk factors for missing the diagnosis of abusive head trauma included younger age, milder symptoms, and social factors such as the child living with two parents and white race. In younger infants, the symptoms of abusive head trauma may be harder to detect because of the immaturity of their nervous systems. With social factors, physicians may be prone to not considering abuse in patients they perceive not to be a risk.

Some infants with fairly mild symptoms such as vomiting, irritability and lethargy could be victims of abusive head trauma. However, these symptoms are so common in infants and toddlers, it is difficult to know which children should have imaging studies of the head and skeletal surveys to look for the diagnosis. Two things might be useful in identifying children at risk. First, a careful 'head to toe' physical examination might reveal other signs of trauma. Second, a dilated retinal examination might reveal retinal haemorrhages. In the future, screening laboratory tests may become available.[42,43] Serum and cerebrospinal fluid markers of brain injury have been identified that appear after traumatic brain injury, including the enzyme neuron-specific enolase, S100B astroglial cell protein, cytochrome c, and quinolinic acid.

Child abuse presents a unique case that may be metabolically different from other types of infant head trauma. First, there often is overwhelming trauma involving all regions of the brain, especially when infants are shaken. Neck injuries in shaken babies may add a unique element that may not be present in accidental injuries. Often there is a delay in seeking care after an inflicted injury, which might worsen the untreated tissue response to injury. Anoxia and uncontrolled cerebral oedema can be a result. Multiple insults over time may confound the severity of injury. Infant brain may be more sensitive and vulnerable to cell death after injury. Levels of neuron-specific enolase were noted to be significantly higher after inflicted traumatic brain injury than after unintentional traumatic brain injury.[43]

PREVENTION

Counselling patients about the dangers of shaking or hitting infants should be part of anticipatory guidance and well-child care. One programme educating new parents about the dangers of shaking infants led to a 50% decrease in the incidence of serious abusive head trauma in the community over a 5-year period (personal communication, Mark Diaz, MD; results currently in press). Home visitation programmes using nurse home visitors have been shown to decrease the incidence of child abuse overall.[44] Child abuse hospitalisation has been shown to be extremely burdensome to society economically.[45] Time and money spent on prevention of abusive head trauma are most likely well worth the cost.

Key points for clinical practice

- Abusive head trauma is difficult to diagnose and often missed.

- Short household falls are not likely to cause serious brain injury.

- Usually, infants experiencing abusive head trauma will become symptomatic shortly after the event occurs.

- Since the term 'shaken baby syndrome' implies a mechanism of injury, the term 'abusive head trauma' might be more precise when the actual mechanism is in question.

- Retinal haemorrhages found in infant abusive head trauma victims are often quite extensive and severe, particularly if the infant has been shaken.

- Victims of abusive head trauma are thought to have a poorer prognosis for neurological recovery than victims of accidental head injuries.

References

1. Barlow KM, Minns RA. Annual incidence of shaken impact syndrome in young children. *Lancet* 2000; **356**: 1571–1572.
2. Jayawant S, Rawlinson A, Gibbon F *et al*. Subdural haemorrhages in infants: population based study. *BMJ* 1998; **317**: 1558–1561.
3. Keenan HT, Runyan DK, Marshall SW, Nocera MA, Merten DF, Sinal SH. A population-based study of inflicted traumatic brain injury in young children. *JAMA* 2003; **290**: 621–626.
4. Keenan HT, Marshall SW, Nocera MA, Runyan DK. Increased incidence of inflicted traumatic brain injury in children after a natural disaster. *Am J Prev Med* 2004; **26**: 189–193.
5. Holbourn AHS. Mechanics of head injuries. *Lancet* 1943; **2**: 438–441.
6. Snyder RG. Impact injury tolerances of infants and children in free falls. Paper presented at 13th Annual Conference of the Association for the Advancement of Automotive Medicine, 1969.
7. Foust DR, Bowan BM, Snyder RG. Study of human impact tolerance using investigations and simulations of free-falls. Paper presented at 21st Stapp Conference, 1977.
8. Ommaya AK, Faas F, Yarnell P. Whiplash injury and brain damage: an experimental study. *JAMA* 1968; **204**: 285–289.
9. Ommaya AK, Hirsch AE. Tolerances for cerebral concussion from head impact and whiplash in primates. *J Biomech* 1971; **4**: 13–21.
10. Gennarelli TA, Thibault LE. Biomechanics of acute subdural hematoma. *J Trauma* 1982; **22**): 680–686.
11. Gennarelli TA, Thibault LE, Adams JH, Graham DI, Thompson CJ, Marcincin RP. Diffuse axonal injury and traumatic coma in the primate. *Ann Neurol* 1982; **12**: 564–574.
12. Adams JH, Gennarelli TA, Graham DI. Brain damage in non-missile head injury: observations in man and subhuman primates. *Rec Adv Neuropathol* 1982; **2**: 165–190.
13. Gennarelli TA, Thibault LE. Directional dependence of axonal brain injury due to centroidal and non-centroidal acceleration. Paper presented at Stapp Conference, 1987.
14. Hymel KP, Bandak FA, Partington MD, Winston KR. Abusive head trauma? A biomechanics-based approach. *Child Maltreatment* 1998; **3**: 116–128.
15. Keenan H. Nomenclature, definitions, incidence, and demographics of inflicted childhood neurotrauma. In: Reece RM, Nicholson CE. (eds) *Inflicted Childhood Neurotrauma*. Elk Grove Village, IL: American Academy of Pediatrics, 2003; 3–16.
16. Duhaime AC, Gennarelli TA, Thibault LE, Bruce DA, Margulies SS, Wiser R. The shaken

baby syndrome. A clinical, pathological, and biomechanical study. *J Neurosurg* 1987; **66**: 409–415.

17. Prange MT, Coats B, Duhaime AC, Margulies SS. Anthropomorphic simulations of falls, shakes, and inflicted impacts in infants. *J Neurosurg* 2003; **99**: 143–150.

18. Cory CZ, Jones BM. Can shaking alone cause fatal brain injury? A biomechanical assessment of the Duhaime shaken baby syndrome model. *Med Sci Law* 2003; **43**: 317–333.

19. American Academy of Paediatrics, Committee on Child Abuse and Neglect. Shaken baby syndrome: rotational cranial injuries-technical report. *Pediatrics* 2001; **108**: 206–210.

20. Alexander R, Sato Y, Smith W, Bennett T. Incidence of impact trauma with cranial injuries ascribed to shaking. *Am J Dis Child* 1990; **144**: 724–726.

21. Atwal GS, Rutty GN, Carter N, Green MA. Bruising in non-accidental head injured children; a retrospective study of the prevalence, distribution and pathological associations in 24 cases. *Forensic Sci Int* 1998; **96**: 215–230.

22. Caffey J. The whiplash shaken infant syndrome: manual shaking by the extremities with whiplash-induced intracranial and intraocular bleedings, linked with residual permanent brain damage and mental retardation. *Pediatrics* 1974; **54**: 396–403.

23. Case ME, Graham MA, Handy TC, Jentzen JM, Monteleone JA. Position paper on fatal abusive head injuries in infants and young children. *Am J Forensic Med Pathol* 2001; **22**: 112–122.

24. Smith C, Bell JE, Keeling JW, Risden RA. Dural haemorrhage in nontraumatic infant deaths: does it explain the bleeding in 'shaken baby syndrome'? Geddes JE *et al*. A response. *Neuropathol Appl Neurobiol* 2003; **29**: 411–412; author reply 412–413.

25. Punt J, Bonshek RE, Jaspan T, McConachie NS, Punt N, Ratcliffe JM. The 'unified hypothesis' of Geddes *et al*. is not supported by the data. *Pediatr Rehabil* 2004; **7**: 173–184.

26. Plunkett J. Fatal pediatric head injuries caused by short-distance falls. *Am J Forensic Med Pathol* 2001; **22**: 1–12.

27. Williams RA. Injuries in infants and small children resulting from witnessed and corroborated free falls. *J Trauma* 1991; **31**: 1350–1352.

28. Musemeche CA, Barthel M, Cosentino C, Reynolds M. Pediatric falls from heights. *J Trauma* 1991; **31**: 1347–1349.

29. Chadwick DL, Chin S, Salerno C, Landsverk J, Kitchen L. Deaths from falls in children: how far is fatal? *J Trauma* 1991; **31**: 1353–1355.

30. Greenwald MJ, Weiss A, Oesterle CS, Friendly DS. Traumatic retinoschisis in battered babies. *Ophthalmology* 1986; **93**: 618–625.

31. Johnson DL, Braun D, Friendly D. Accidental head trauma and retinal hemorrhage. *Neurosurgery* 1993; **33**: 231–234; discussion 234–235.

32. Gilliland MG, Luckenbach MW, Chenier TC. Systemic and ocular findings in 169 prospectively studied child deaths: retinal hemorrhages usually mean child abuse. *Forensic Sci Int* 1994; **68**: 117–132.

33. Levin AV. Ophthalmology of shaken baby syndrome. *Neurosurg Clin North Am* 2002; **13**: 201–211, vi.

34. Morad Y, Kim YM, Armstrong DC, Huyer D, Mian M, Levin AV. Correlation between retinal abnormalities and intracranial abnormalities in the shaken baby syndrome. *Am J Ophthalmol* 2002; **134**: 354–359.

35. Ewing-Cobbs L, Kramer L, Prasad M *et al*. Neuroimaging, physical, and developmental findings after inflicted and noninflicted traumatic brain injury in young children. *Pediatrics* 1998; **102**: 300–307.

36. Reece RM, Sege R. Childhood head injuries: accidental or inflicted? *Arch Pediatr Adolesc Med* 2000; **154**: 11–15.

37. Michaud LJ. Inflicted childhood neurotrauma: Outcomes and rehabilitation. In: Reece RM, Nicholson CE. (eds) *Inflicted Childhood Neurotrauma*. Elk Grove Village, IL: American Academy of Pediatrics, 2003; 255–264.

38. Willman KY, Bank DE, Senac M, Chadwick DL. Restricting the time of injury in fatal inflicted head injuries. *Child Abuse Negl* 1997; **21**: 929–940.

39. Humphreys RP, Hendrick EB, Hoffman HJ. The head-injured child who 'talks and dies'. A report of 4 cases. *Child Nerv Syst* 1990; **6**: 139–142.

40. Starling SP, Patel S, Burke BL, Sirotnak AP, Stronks S, Rosquist P. Analysis of perpetrator

admissions to inflicted traumatic brain injury in children. *Arch Pediatr Adolesc Med* 2004; **158**: 454–458.

41. Jenny C, Hymel KP, Ritzen A, Reinert SE, Hay TC. Analysis of missed cases of abusive head trauma. *JAMA* 1999; **281**: 621–626.

42. Berger RP, Pierce MC, Wisniewski SR, Adelson PD, Kochanek PM. Serum S100B concentrations are increased after closed head injury in children: a preliminary study. *J Neurotrauma* 2002; **19**: 1405–1409.

43. Berger RP, Pierce MC, Wisniewski SR *et al*. Neuron-specific enolase and S100B in cerebrospinal fluid after severe traumatic brain injury in infants and children. *Pediatrics* 2002; **109**: E31.

44. Olds DL, Henderson Jr CR, Chamberlin R, Tatelbaum R. Preventing child abuse and neglect: a randomized trial of nurse home visitation. *Pediatrics* 1986; **78**: 65–78.

45. Rovi S, Chen PH, Johnson MS. The economic burden of hospitalizations associated with child abuse and neglect. *Am J Public Health* 2004; **94**: 586–590.

Peter Sidebotham Peter Fleming Peter Blair

2

Sudden unexpected death in infancy

Every year in the UK, over 300 babies die suddenly and unexpectedly.[1] Each one of these deaths is a tragedy for the families involved and leaves the parents bewildered and confused, inevitably asking that dreadful question 'Why?' Sadly, for many parents there will be no answer. For some, there will be an identifiable reason for their baby's death; for others, a thorough investigation will fail to find a specific cause. In a small minority, one or both parents may have contributed to their child's death, either deliberately or inadvertently. Whatever the underlying reasons, all parents will experience feelings of grief and loss, and most too will feel some sense of responsibility or guilt.

As paediatricians, we have a responsibility to parents that extends beyond their baby's death. We can offer support and advice, and most importantly, we can play a crucial role in investigating the death, and where possible, identifying causal or contributory factors. But we cannot do so alone. All infant deaths deserve the fullest evaluation, including a thorough history, a comprehensive review of the circumstances of the death (including consideration of the possibilities of both natural and unnatural events), and a thorough post mortem examination, to an agreed evidence-based protocol. Sadly, all too often, the traumatic experience these families have been through is further compounded by insensitive or incomplete investigations and support.

Peter Sidebotham MB ChB MRCP MSc (for correspondence)
Senior Lecturer in Child Health, Warwick Medical School, University of Warwick, Coventry CV4 7AL, UK
E-mail: p.sidebotham@bristol.ac.uk

Peter Fleming PhD MB ChB FRCP(Lond) FRCP(Can) FRCPH
Professor of Infant Health and Developmental Physiology, University of Bristol and Consultant Paediatrician, United Bristol Healthcare NHS Trust, Bristol, UK

Peter Blair MSc PhD
Medical Statistician, Division of Child Health, University of Bristol, Education Centre, Upper Maudlin Street, Bristol BS2 8AE, UK

In this chapter, we will outline factors contributing to sudden unexpected death in infancy (SUDI), showing how a thorough, co-ordinated approach to investigation and management can be effective in identifying such factors. We review the epidemiology and recognised risk factors for SUDI; summarise some of the causes of sudden death in infancy, and provide some pointers for distinguishing natural from unnatural sudden deaths. We will focus on sudden infant death syndrome (SIDS) as those deaths which remain unexplained following a thorough case investigation, and will provide an update on current understanding of the possible mechanisms for SIDS. Finally, we will outline our current practice in the joint agency management of SUDI, an approach which has been recommended for national adoption[2] and which we believe is practical, evidence based, and achievable.[3]

EPIDEMIOLOGY OF SUDI

During the 1990s, many countries experienced a dramatic fall in the incidence of SUDI (Fig. 1). Prior to 1988, the rate was about 2 per 1000 live births in the UK. This dropped by 1995 to 0.61 per 1000.[4] Since then, the rate has been stable with just a slow decline to 0.48 per 1000 in 2002. The decline has almost entirely been related to a fall in the number of SIDS deaths, whilst the number of explained SUDI (including abuse-related SUDI) has remained stable (Table 1). Nevertheless, SIDS remains the commonest cause of death in the postneonatal period, accounting for 28% of such deaths in 2002.[1]

Many of the epidemiological features that characterise SIDS infants and their families have remained the same, despite the fall in incidence. These

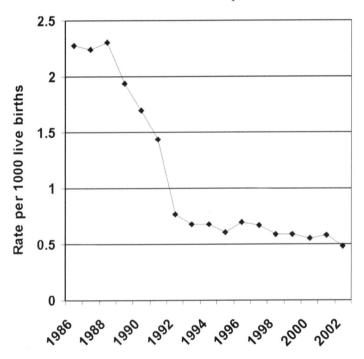

Fig. 1 Sudden infant deaths, England and Wales 1986–2002.

Table 1 Changing epidemiology of SUDI

	Incidence of SIDS	incidence of explained SUDI	Incidence of NAI as a cause of SUDI
1985–1991	1:428	1:3650	1:17,000
1992–1998	1:2650	1:3750	1:15,000
1999–2003	1:1430	1:2350	1:16,000

Data from the Avon Infant Mortality Study.
NAI, non-accidental injury.

include the characteristic age distribution, with few deaths in the first few weeks of life or after 6 months and a peak between 10 and 16 weeks; a higher incidence in males; lower birthweight; a shorter gestation and more problems at delivery. There is a strong correlation with young maternal age and higher parity and the risk increases for infants of single mothers and for multiple births. A small, but significant, proportion of mothers have also experienced a previous stillbirth or infant death. SIDS occurs in all social strata but is more prevalent amongst poorer families. The majority of SIDS deaths still occur during the night sleep and in studies in the UK there has been no particular day of the week with consistently increased prevalence.

Major epidemiological features to change include a reduction in the previous high winter peaks of death and a shift of SIDS families to the more deprived social grouping. The strongest identified environmental risk factor remains exposure to tobacco smoke, both prenatal and postnatal, with a clear biological gradient of increased risk with increased exposure. However, these background epidemiological factors are not unique to SIDS, and many are common amongst infants who die from other causes.[5] Only the age profile and parental smoking distinguish SIDS infants from other infant deaths.

UNDERSTANDING RISK FACTORS

For some epidemiological factors (*e.g.* poverty, preterm delivery, low birthweight) a clear relationship with SIDS can be demonstrated, but the nature of that relationship and ways in which it might be amenable to intervention have not been identified. For others (*e.g.* tobacco exposure) the relationship is sufficiently strong to be considered causal, but the mechanism is unclear and interventions have so far been ineffective. It is perhaps in the infant sleeping environment that the epidemiological study of SIDS has had the most success. Studies since 1991 have shown that the previously common practice of placing infants to sleep on their front has almost disappeared (now < 3% compared to 90% during the 1980s). The initial campaigns suggested the side position as a safe alternative although it has since been found this position carries a significant risk, mainly because young infants who roll from side to prone may be unable to extricate themselves from this position.[6] Other risk factors in the sleeping environment include the potential for both heat stress and head covering which inspired the 'Feet to Foot' campaign advising parents

Table 2 Advice on reducing the risks

Encourage
- Supine sleeping position for infants
- Placing the infant in the 'feet to foot' position
- Sharing a room with the baby for the first 6 months
- Immunisation

Discourage
- Exposure of pregnant women and infants to cigarette smoke
- Sleeping with the infant on a sofa or armchair
- Bed-sharing when parents are smokers, are tired or have taken alcohol/drugs to help sleep
- Heavy wrapping and high room temperature
- Pillows, duvets or loose bedding

to place the cot next to the parental bed, the feet of the infant at the foot of the cot, to avoid duvets or pillows and to use thin layers of covering firmly tucked in. (Foundation for the Study of Infant deaths. BabyZone leaflet. E-mail: fsid@sids.org.uk; or visit the website: <http://www.sids.org.uk/fsis/fsid>.)

More recent studies have found other significant risk factors within the infant sleeping environment although the advice related to these is not so clear-cut. For instance, there has been increasing evidence that infants who habitually use a dummy, but do not do so on a particular night, are more at risk of SIDS.[7,8] Another factor under much debate is the risk associated with bed-sharing. Recent studies have shown an increase in prevalence of bed-sharing SIDS from 10–15% prior to the 1991 campaign to 40–50% after.[9,10] Examination of the longitudinal data suggests the actual number of SIDS deaths in the parental bed has gone down, albeit not to the same dramatic extent as SIDS occurring in a solitary cot environment. One of the reasons for this change may be that placing bed-sharing infants prone to sleep has always been less common so that any intervention campaign would have less impact on this group of infants. There may also have been an increase in the number of SIDS infants found co-sleeping with a parent on a sofa (where entrapment is often suspected but not proven). Alcohol consumption and heavy adult duvets have been implicated as possible confounders[11] and the risk of bed-sharing appears to be mainly limited to younger infants (< 4 months) and parents who smoke.

In the light of our current understanding,[12] some clear messages can be given to parents on how to reduce the risks of cot death, most notably to encourage the supine and 'feet to foot' sleeping position, and to discourage exposure of infants and pregnant women to cigarette smoke (Table 2). Other risks, such as those relating to bed sharing cannot be summarised with a simplistic message; rather, we need to highlight the particular circumstances that put such infants at risk.

CAUSES OF SUDDEN DEATH IN INFANCY

With the fall in the overall prevalence of sudden infant deaths, a greater proportion of these are now found to have an identifiable cause. The CESDI studies of 1993–1996 identified 93 explained deaths out of a total 456 SUDI

(20%).[13] The commonest identified causes were infection (38%), trauma (39%) and (previously unrecognised) congenital malformations (11%). A further 5% were due to gastrointestinal conditions and 4% to metabolic disorders. It is interesting that the epidemiological profile of these explained deaths is very similar to that of SIDS, with a winter peak, social deprivation, young maternal age, smoking, low birthweight and prematurity.[13] The major difference is that more of these explained deaths occur in the first month of life.

INFECTIONS

Infections, particularly meningococcal or pneumococcal disease, can progress very rapidly in both infants and older children and make up the largest group of medical causes. Septicaemia, meningitis, myocarditis, encephalitis, broncho-pneumonia, bronchiolitis and peritonitis have all been identified in SUDI.

Myocarditis may be caused by a wide variety of viruses and other infectious agents, and may show little more than non-specific clinical signs. Diagnosis is dependent on the finding of an inflammatory cell infiltrate with myocyte necrosis and may be supported by the finding of micro-organisms in blood or cardiac tissue.[14] Upper respiratory tract infections including croup and epiglottitis may lead to sudden death, although typically there will be some antecedent symptoms, and the incidence of epiglottitis has dropped substantially with the introduction of *Haemophilus influenzae* B immunisation. The incidence of pertussis has also dropped due to immunisation, but it may still present in infancy with sudden death due to apnoea. Much more common are lower respiratory tract infections including bronchopneumonia and bronchiolitis. In both of these, preceding symptoms may be mild and non-specific. Respiratory infections are, however, extremely common and most infants recover completely, even when radiology reveals gross changes on the lungs. Many infants with significant pulmonary infiltrates and/or consolidation present with varying degrees of respiratory distress, but survive. Thus, the finding of intrapulmonary pathology may reflect a contributory factor in a compromised infant rather than a complete and sufficient explanation for the death.[14]

Meningitis may present in infancy with a rapid course and minimal or non-specific symptoms. *H. influenzae*, *Staphylococcus pneumoniae* and *Neisseria meningitidis* are the commonest infecting organisms, along with Group B Streptococci and enterobacteria in the neonatal period. A rapidly fulminating course may result in fatal septicaemia before the onset of meningitis and the lethal effects are thought to be due to circulating endotoxins. These endotoxins may lead to pathological changes to the myocardium and adrenal glands that can be picked up at autopsy. *Staphylococcus aureus* may also cause sudden death in infants due to release of systemically acting toxins. The diagnosis of lethal septicaemia is dependent on positive blood cultures and/or isolation of the same organism from multiple sites, preferably with microscopic evidence of disseminated sepsis.[14]

CARDIOVASCULAR CAUSES

Sudden death has been reported in a wide range of congenital heart defects arising *de novo*, or following cardiac surgery. Causes of death in these situations include fatal arrhythmias, cardiac failure, infarction and endocarditis.[14] One case series found associated cardiac disease in 9.7% of sudden unexpected infant deaths.[15] In 60% of these deaths, the diagnosis had not been recognised before autopsy. Cardiomyopathy, both primary and secondary to metabolic disorders, may result in sudden death, as may endocardial fibroelastosis. Whilst a range of cardiac arrhythmias may account for sudden death, the most commonly quoted are the long QT syndromes.[16] Specific syndromes with recognised genetic mutations have been described and linked to sudden infant deaths. Since conduction defects cannot be identified at autopsy, the diagnosis must rest on the clinical and family history and appropriate molecular studies.

GASTROINTESTINAL CAUSES

Fulminant gastroenteritis with severe dehydration and electrolyte imbalance may lead to death from cardiac arrhythmias, cerebral haemorrhage or venous thrombosis. Clinical signs may be apparent at autopsy, and analysis of vitreous humour may reveal electrolyte imbalances. Other gastrointestinal conditions, including intestinal obstruction may occasionally present as sudden death, but will usually be obvious at autopsy.[14] Gastro-oesophageal reflux has been suggested as a possible cause of SIDS, through vagally mediated apnoea. Strong evidence in support of this theory is lacking, however, and it is unlikely to account for more than a small proportion of these deaths.

METABOLIC DISORDERS

Inborn errors of metabolism represent a disparate group of disorders, all of which are individually rare, but which in total may account for a substantial proportion of SUDI.[14] Features in the history that may point to an underlying metabolic disorder include failure to thrive, developmental delay, seizures, and vomiting and diarrhoea. An enlarged liver or spleen may be noted on examination; at autopsy, cardiomegaly, cerebral oedema and fatty changes in the liver, kidneys and muscle may be found. However, these changes are not specific to metabolic disorders and may be found, for example, in acute dehydration and severe infection. The commonest metabolic defects to present this way are the disorders of fatty acid oxidation, particularly deficiencies of acyl CoA dehydrogenases, both medium-chain (MCAD) and, less commonly, long-chain (LCAD). In these disorders, episodic hypoglycaemia, encephalopathy and respiratory depression with apnoea may be precipitated by viral illness or by fasting. Sudden deaths have also been reported in glycogen storage diseases, mitochondrial respiratory chain defects, amino acid disorders and other rare disorders.[14]

TRAUMA

Deaths due to major trauma will usually be apparent from the history, examination or autopsy, and include deaths from intracranial haemorrhage, abdominal trauma with ruptured organs, and multiple trauma. Asphyxia, both accidental and inflicted may be less easy to detect. Features that may help to distinguish accidental from intentional deaths are outlined below (sudden deaths due to child maltreatment).

SUDDEN INFANT DEATH SYNDROME

SIDS remains the largest group of unexpected deaths in infancy. The diagnosis is one of exclusion and should be used according to stringent criteria. The commonest accepted definition is 'the sudden death of an infant under one year of age which remains unexplained after a thorough case investigation, including performance of a complete autopsy, examination of the death scene and review of the clinical history'.[17] Typically, babies dying of SIDS will be found by their parents in the morning lying in their beds where they had been put down. There will often be a history of minor illness in the 48 h preceding the death and it is common for the GP to have been consulted in that time. At autopsy, various characteristic findings have been identified, including petechial haemorrhages of thymus, pleura and epicardium. However, these findings are neither diagnostic nor obligatory and may be found in both natural and unnatural deaths.[18]

PATHOGENESIS OF SIDS: ELUSIVE PATHWAYS

In spite of considerable advances in our understanding of the epidemiology of SIDS and of factors affecting risk, we are little closer to understanding why babies die suddenly and unexpectedly where no causal factor is found. There is some evidence that 'the fatal event involves a neurally-compromised infant, circumstances that challenge vital physiology, most likely during sleep, at a particular developmental period'.[19]

The effects of prenatal exposure to tobacco smoke, along with other antenatal risk factors suggest that those infants who later succumb to SIDS may in some ways be compromised from an early stage. The recently reported association with elevated maternal α-fetoprotein in the second trimester would also support this suggestion.[20] It is possible that these infants may have enhanced arousal thresholds and be less able to respond through normal homeostatic mechanisms to particular environmental challenges. Changes in normal arousal have been shown in infants at risk for SIDS.[21]

Two key pathways have been proposed to account for the impact of sleeping position and environment on risk of SIDS.[12] First, sleeping position may affect respiratory control, through re-breathing of expired gases or through direct suffocation, either from bedding, or in the case of co-sleeping, from proximity to a parent. Second, the adverse effects of heat stress from ambient temperature, heavy wrapping, head coverings or proximity to others. It is postulated that thermal stress might lead to death through the direct effects of raised temperature on sensitive central neural processes, or by effects on other homeostatic mechanisms.[22]

As research knowledge and standardised, evidence-based investigation increases, it is likely that a greater number of cases of SUDI will have an identifiable cause. In particular, further advances in genetics and metabolic studies may reveal specific factors that lead to the infant vulnerability alluded to above. However, it is extremely unlikely that SIDS as such will ever yield to a single causal pathway, but is more likely to be a reflection of a variety of causes and contributory factors.

SUDDEN DEATH DUE TO MALTREATMENT

Although the vast majority of sudden, unexpected deaths in infancy arise from natural (though not necessarily well understood) causes, a significant proportion occur as a direct or indirect result of child maltreatment. Whilst some cases of homicide will be obvious, most are difficult to recognise, with no specific features, and many probably go unrecognised. Estimates of the proportion of SUDI caused by homicide vary considerably,[23] although many authors suggest up to 10% may be frank homicide, with maltreatment (abuse or neglect) being a contributory (though not necessarily causal) factor in a similar proportion. In the CESDI SUDI study of 456 SUDI in 1993–1996, maltreatment was thought to be the main cause of death for a total of 25 infants (6.0%), and a secondary or alternative cause of death for a further 32 infants (7.7%).[24] In our experience there are often features in the history or scene examination that suggest poor care, though not sufficient to warrant consideration of abuse or neglect.

Deaths due to maltreatment may arise as a result of inflicted injury, suffocation, poisoning, or gross neglect. Cases of inflicted injury include intracranial injury due to shaking, abdominal trauma, and multiple trauma. In most cases, the diagnosis will become apparent through the history and gross post mortem findings. However, cases of shaken baby syndrome may be subtle with no external or internal injuries other than the intracranial trauma. Gross neglect may lead to death through starvation, hypothermia, or in association with other forms of maltreatment. In most cases, examination findings will raise suspicions and there will often have been pre-existing concerns about the family. Poisoning may not be apparent from the history or gross pathology, although biochemical studies may provide some clues. Some investigators have recommended the routine use of toxicology in the investigation of SUDI,[25,26] although the overall positive yield is low.

Perhaps the most difficult differential diagnosis in SUDI cases is that between SIDS and either accidental or intentional asphyxiation. Although findings such as alveolar haemorrhages may be found in cases of suffocation, these findings are not specific. Similarly, the presence of blood around the nose and mouth may raise concerns but again is not diagnostic. It is important to distinguish the finding of frank blood (which is relatively rare) from the very common finding of frothy, blood-stained fluid around the nose and mouth. The finding of haemosiderin-laden macrophages in the lung has been reported in association with possible previous episodes of asphyxia, but gives no indication of the cause. Cases of accidental asphyxiation due to entrapment or overlaying may be apparent from the history or the scene examination. Deliberate suffocation, through the use of a soft object such as a pillow is impossible to identify from pathological examination.

In seeking to distinguish SIDS from death due to maltreatment, a number of characteristics may raise suspicions. The American Academy of Pediatrics[26] suggests that the possibility of maltreatment should be considered in the following circumstances:

- Previous recurrent cyanosis, apnoea, or apparent life-threatening episodes while in the care of the same person

- Age at death older than 6 months

- Previous unexpected or unexplained deaths of 1 or more siblings

- Simultaneous or nearly simultaneous death of twins

- Previous death of infants under the care of the same unrelated person

- Discovery of blood on the infant's nose or mouth in association with apparent life-threatening episodes.

It is important to recognise that none of these findings are diagnostic of maltreatment, and in most instances no clear evidence of maltreatment will emerge. It is important that each finding should be carefully interpreted in the light of the full clinical picture.

A history of previous unexplained illness, including apparent life-threatening episodes (ALTEs) has been found in cases of fabricated and induced illness, but also in many infants who die as SIDS. If such a history is forthcoming, previous records should be checked and a careful history taken, to include details of who was present on each occasion. However, isolated brief episodes of apparent lifelessness may be quite common in the general population and recurrent episodes may be an indicator of underlying cardiovascular, respiratory, neurological or metabolic disease. In the CESDI SUDI study, 11.7% of SIDS victims and 3% of control infants were noted to have experienced one or more such episodes.[24]

The age at death is perhaps one of strongest indicators. SIDS cases show a distinct age-profile with a peak at 2–3 months, and most cases occurring before 6 months. Deaths in the first month are more likely to be due to underlying medical factors, whilst unexplained deaths from natural causes are proportionately less likely over the age of 6 months. Deaths outside the age range of 6 weeks to 6 months should prompt an even more thorough search for underlying medical or forensic explanations.

Previous unexpected or unexplained deaths in siblings have been the subject of much controversy. The much-quoted rule of thumb – 'one sudden infant death is a tragedy, two is suspicious, three is murder until proved otherwise' – is dangerously simplistic and potentially misleading. Perhaps a far better rule of thumb is that in any case of repeated unexpected deaths there is likely to be some underlying explanation for the deaths, whether medical, forensic or environmental.

MANAGEMENT OF SUDI

In the investigation and management of sudden deaths several parallel needs must be fulfilled. First, the family's needs must be recognised – including the need for information and support. There is: (i) a need to identify any underlying medical causes of death that may have genetic or public health implications; (ii) a legal need for a thorough forensic investigation to exclude unnatural causes of death; and (iii) the need to protect siblings and subsequent children. Alongside this, there is the need to protect families from false or

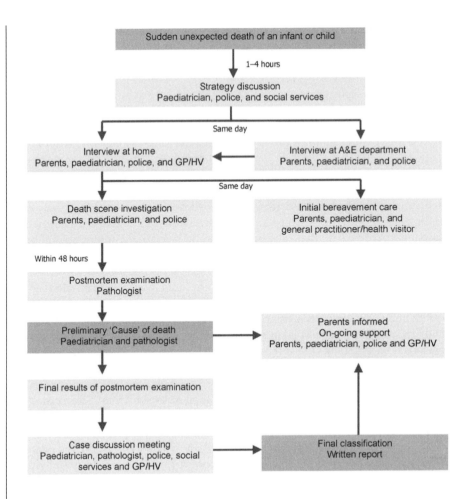

Fig. 2 The Avon and Somerset approach to the management of sudden unexpected deaths in childhood.

inappropriate accusations, to investigate the death thoroughly whilst remaining sensitive to the needs of the family at a very difficult time.

Any approach to the management of SUDI must recognise these conflicting needs and be based on a thorough understanding of recent research. The following outline (Fig. 2) describes the approach used in Avon and Somerset.[3] It is important to remember that, as in most of medicine, the single most useful component of the investigation of SUDI is a very detailed clinical history, which should include a detailed description of the precise circumstances of the death.[27]

INITIAL AMBULANCE RESPONSE AND MANAGEMENT IN THE EMERGENCY DEPARTMENT

In almost all cases of sudden unexpected death, the parents' first response is to call an ambulance. The ambulance crew will normally commence resuscitation and transfer the baby with one or both parents to the emergency department, where the hospital staff will further assess the baby and continue or cease resuscitation as appropriate. In the emergency department, a named nurse is allocated to the family on arrival and will be the main point of liaison and support throughout the initial stages. Sensitivity to the family's needs is paramount at all stages, and with this in mind, the baby is always referred to by name, the family are allowed to hold their baby as much as they wish, and mementoes and photographs are taken. A minimum of investigations should be undertaken in the emergency department, but if resuscitation is attempted, blood should be taken at the time for glucose and electrolyte analysis, and for culture. We do not recommend cardiac puncture as this can compromise the subsequent autopsy. Most sampling can safely be left to the post mortem, but any samples taken should be carefully labelled and stored for further analysis if required. If there is a history suggestive of possible metabolic disorder, an early frozen section of liver can be invaluable.

EARLY STRATEGIC DISCUSSION

As soon as possible after every sudden unexpected infant death, a strategic discussion is held involving the paediatrician, the police child protection team and the social services duty team. The purpose of the discussion is to plan how best to investigate the death and to support the family. At this initial discussion, basic information is shared, initial checks of the family are carried out and decisions are made as to which professionals will see the family and at what stage. In all cases, arrangements will be made for a joint home visit by the paediatrician and police officer, along with the GP or health visitor. These visits usually take place within a few hours of the death.

JOINT HOME VISIT BY POLICE AND PAEDIATRICIAN

The purposes of the home visit are 3-fold: (i) to start the investigation, gathering information from the history and examination of the scene of death; (ii) to inform the family of the process of the investigation, and provide information; and (iii) to ensure that support is available to the family. We have found that by being clear about the need for a joint agency approach and about the different aspects that will be covered in the investigation, families seem to be appreciative and find the joint visits to be helpful rather than intrusive. A full medical and social history is taken, with particular emphasis on recent events. The parents are given time to talk through the events leading up to the death, as well as the background history of their baby and a wider review of the family and home circumstances. Whilst a narrative approach is taken, allowing the family to take the lead and go at their own place, the recording of the history is structured to ensure that all aspects are covered (Box 1).

Different approaches to the death scene investigation have previously been described.[28,29] Our approach involves taking a video, using a structured format to ensure that all aspects of the environment are captured. In most cases, one of the parents will talk through the final events, demonstrating where and how the baby was lying when put down and when found. We have found that this approach ensures that we obtain a very thorough understanding of the circumstances around the death, have been able to inform the pathologist of

---

Box 1 Structured approach to the initial interview

1. Basic details of baby, the parents and other family members

2. A narrative account of the 24 hours leading up to the baby's death

   This should include a full description of when and how the baby slept and fed, any activity, who was with the baby at different times, the baby's health and activity levels, any changes to routine.

3. The final sleep

   Where and how the baby was put down, clothing, bed coverings, position; any changes in that during the course of the night; if bed sharing, who else was in the bed and their positions relative to the baby; when and by whom the baby was checked during the sleep; description of the last feed and any night time feeds; heating and ventilation.

   Where and how the baby was found, position, coverings, appearance and any unusual features; any action taken after the baby was found.

4. Baby's past medical history

   Including pregnancy and delivery, growth and development, feeding, any illnesses, immunisations and routine surveillance. Also details of normal routine for the baby, including feeding and sleeping patterns and practices.

5. Family medical history

   Including any medical or psychiatric history of the parents and other immediate family members. Any previous infant deaths in the family.

6. Social history

   Family structure and dynamics, housing, use of alcohol, recreational drugs and tobacco. Parents' occupations. Any social services involvement in the past, including any child protection concerns.

---

specific factors to look for, and in many cases have been able to offer reassurance to the family about the manner in which their child died.

POST MORTEM EXAMINATION

A full post mortem examination is conducted to an agreed protocol. Various protocols have been described previously and we have built on these, using an evidence-based approach that balances the probability of obtaining useful information against the needs of parents for the examination to be completed quickly, with a minimum of tissue retention.[2,24]

Following the post mortem, the pathologist will, in consultation with the paediatrician, ascertain a cause of death to be fed back to the coroner and, following discussion with the multi-agency team, to the family. This will often involve a second home visit with a member of the primary care team.

In the small number of cases where child protection concerns are identified, there will be a more formal multi-agency strategy meeting under Section 47 of the *Children Act*. Consideration will be given at that meeting to how any criminal or child protection investigation will be carried out, any on-going needs for other children in the family, what support the family will need during the course of the investigation, and what information can be given to the family and by whom.

Classification**	0	I A	I B	II A	II B	III
Contributory or potentially 'causal' Factors	Information not collected	No factors identified	Present but not likely to have contributed to ill health or to death.	Present, and may have contributed to ill health, or possibly to death	Present and certainly contributed to ill health, and probably contributed to the death	Present, and provides a complete and sufficient cause of death
Social factors						
Non-accidental injury/ evidence of abuse or harm						
Past Medical history						
Family history						
History of final events						
Death-scene examination						
Radiology						
Toxicology						
Microbiology / Virology						
Gross pathology						
Histology						
Biochemistry						
Metabolic investigations						
Special investigations (e.g. histochemistry)						
Other (specify)						
Overall classification **						

** *This will equal the highest individual classification listed above. NB an entry (0, I, II, or III) MUST be made on every line of the grid.*

Fig. 3 The Avon clinicopathological classification of SUDI.

MULTI-AGENCY CASE DISCUSSION MEETING

At 2–3 months after the death, a case discussion meeting is held, involving all professionals who were involved with the family. This gives an opportunity to review all aspects of the investigation, to consider any causal or contributory factors that have been identified (Fig. 3), and to plan for continuing support of the family. It also gives an opportunity to debrief those involved in the care of the family, recognising the emotional cost of dealing with such deaths. Information from the multi-agency case discussion meeting is also given to the coroner, and will inform the conduct and outcome of the inquest.[2]

The meeting is followed by a final visit to the family by the paediatrician and GP or health visitor to feed back the findings from the full investigation, to review how things have gone since their baby's death, and to talk through any ongoing support needs.

CARE OF FUTURE INFANTS

Any family who has experienced an infant death will inevitably experience concerns about the safety of future children. In order to minimise these concerns, and support the family in any steps they take to reduce the risks, it is important to offer comprehensive follow-up of future infants. In many parts of the country this is carried out through the CONI (Care of the Next Infant) scheme (<www.sids.org.uk/fsid/coni>). The key components of this care are advice to the family during pregnancy, training in infant resuscitation, advice on reducing the risks, regular review by a paediatrician, frequent health visitor contact with regular weighing of the baby, and clear contact details for the family in case of concerns. Whilst apnoea monitors or more complex cardiorespiratory or oxygenation monitors have not been shown to be of any direct value in preventing further infant deaths,[30] some families find their use re-assuring. For many families, however, the frequent false alarms from such devices add to their anxiety rather than helping.

Although there is undoubtedly an increased risk of death in subsequent babies, this risk remains low (< 1%) and parents can be re-assured. The sudden unexpected death of an infant is perhaps the worst experience any family can go through, and takes its toll on all involved. However, to see a healthy thriving infant make it through the first year, especially when the family has been able to modify previously identified risks, is one of the most rewarding experiences for any professional working in the field.

Key points for clinical practice

- In spite of significant reductions in incidence in the early 1990s, SIDS remains the commonest cause of postneonatal deaths.

- SIDS accounts for up to 70% of sudden unexpected deaths in infancy and is a diagnosis of exclusion. The term should be used strictly to refer to the sudden death of an infant under 1 year of age which remains unexplained after a thorough case investigation, including performance of a complete autopsy, examination of the death scene and review of the clinical history. Unless and until those criteria are fulfilled, deaths should be referred to as sudden unexpected deaths in infancy.

- With appropriate and thorough investigation, a cause can be found for at least 30% of SUDI; the commonest causes being infectious disease, metabolic disease and trauma.

- Fatal child abuse accounts for up to 10% of SUDI. In a similar proportion, there may be evidence of sub-optimal care.

- The risks of SUDI can be reduced by placing infants supine in the 'feet to foot' position; by infants sharing a room with their parents for the first 6 months; by avoiding exposure of pregnant women and children to cigarette smoke; by avoiding heavy wrapping and high room temperatures; and by avoiding bed sharing when parents are smokers, are tired or have taken alcohol or sleep-inducing drugs.

- The investigation of all SUDI should be through a multi-agency approach involving a thorough detailed history; a joint paediatric/police visit to the home with examination of the scene; and a comprehensive post mortem examination. This should be followed up after 2–3 months, by a case discussion meeting to draw together the different elements of the investigation, in order to classify the death, identify any contributory factors and plan for continuing support for the family.

References

1. Office for National Statistics. *Deaths 2002: Childhood, infant and perinatal mortality: live births, stillbirths and linked infant deaths by ONS cause groups and mother's country of birth.* 2002, London: Office for National Statistics, 2002; <http://www.statistics.gov.uk/STATBASE/>.
2. Anon. *Sudden Unexpected Death in Infancy.* London: The Royal College of Pathologists and The Royal College of Paediatrics and Child Health, 2004; <www.rcpath.org>.
3. Fleming PJ, Blair P, Sidebotham P, Hayler T. Investigating sudden unexpected deaths in infancy and childhood and caring for bereaved families: an integrated multiagency approach. *BMJ* 2004; **328**: 331–334.
4. Office for National Statistics. *ONS Monitor Population and Health DH3 series: Sudden infant deaths.* London: Office for National Statistics, 1996.
5. Leach CEA, Blair PS, Fleming PJ *et al.* Sudden unexpected deaths in infancy: similarities and differences in the epidemiology of SIDS and explained deaths. *Pediatrics* 1999; **104**: 43–52.
6. Fleming PJ, Blair PS, Bacon C *et al.* Environment of infants during sleep and risk of the sudden infant death syndrome: results from 1993–5 case-control study for confidential inquiry into stillbirths and deaths in infancy. *BMJ* 1996; **313**: 191–195.
7. Mitchell EA, Taylor BJ, Ford RPK *et al.* Dummies and the sudden infant death syndrome. *Arch Dis Child* 1993; **68**: 501–504.
8. Fleming PJ, Blair PS, Pollard K *et al.* Pacifier use and sudden infant death syndrome: results from the CESDI/SUDI case control study. *Arch Dis Child* 1999; **81**: 112–116.
9. Carpenter PR, Irgens PL, Blair PS *et al.* Sudden unexplained infant death in 20 regions in Europe: case control study. *Lancet* 2004; **363**: 185–191.

10. McGarvey C, McDonnell M, Chong A, O'Regan M, Matthews T. Factors relating to the infant's last sleep environment in sudden infant death syndrome in the Republic of Ireland. *Arch Dis Child* 2003; **88**: 1058–1064.

11. Blair PS, Fleming PJ, Smith IJ *et al* and the CESDI SUDI Research Group. Babies sleeping with parents: case-control study of factors influencing the risk of sudden infant death syndrome. *BMJ* 1999; **319**: 1457–1462.

12. American Academy of Pediatrics. Changing concepts of sudden infant death syndrome: implications for infant sleeping environment and sleeping position. *Pediatrics* 2000; **105**: 650–656.

13. Maternal and Child Health Research Consortium. *CESDI 5th Annual Report, 1998.* London: Maternal and Child Health Research Consortium, 1998; <www.cesdi.org.uk/publications>.

14. Byard RW. *Sudden Death in Infancy, Childhood and Adolescence,* 2nd edn. Cambridge: Cambridge University Press, 2004.

15. Danacea A, Cote A, Robliceck C, Bernard C, Oligny L. Cardiac pathology in sudden unexpected infant death. *J Pediatr* 2002; **141**: 336–342.

16. Schwartz PJ, Priori SG, Dumaine R *et al.* A molecular link between the sudden infant death syndrome and the long-QT interval. *N Engl J Med* 2000; **343**: 262–267.

17. Willinger M, James LS, Catz C. Defining the sudden infant death syndrome (SIDS): deliberations of an expert panel convened by the National Institute of Child Health and Human Development. *Pediatr Pathol* 1991; **11**: 677–684.

18. Byard RW, Krous HF. Sudden infant death syndrome: overview and update. *Pediatr Dev Pathol* 2003; **6**: 112–127.

19. Harper RM, Kinney HC, Fleming PJ, Thach BT. Sleep influences on homeostatic functions: implications for sudden infant death syndrome. *Respir Physiol* 2000; **119**: 123–132.

20. Smith GC, Wood AM, Pell JP, White IR, Crossley JA, Dobbie R. Second trimester maternal serum levels of alpha-fetoprotein and the subsequent risk of SIDS. *N Engl J Med* 2004; **351**: 978–986.

21. Newman NM, Trinder JA, Phillips KA, Jordan K, Cruickshank J. Arousal deficit: mechanism of the sudden infant death syndrome? *Aust Paediatr J* 1989; **25**: 196–201.

22. Fleming PJ, Levine MR, Azaz Y, Wigfield R. The development of thermoregulation and interactions with the control of respiration in infants: possible relationship to sudden infant death. *Acta Paediatr Scand* 1993; **Suppl 389**: 57–59.

23. Levene S, Bacon C. Sudden unexpected death and covert homicide. *Arch Dis Child* 2004; **89**: 443–447.

24. Fleming PJ, Blair P, Bacon C, Berry PJ. *Sudden Unexpected Deaths in Infancy. The CESDI SUDI Studies 1993–1996.* London: The Stationery Office: London, 2000.

25. Arnestad M, Vege A, Rognum T. Evaluation of diagnostic tools applied in the examination of sudden unexpected deaths in infancy and early childhood. *Forensic Sci Int* 2002; **125**: 262–268.

26. American Academy of Pediatrics. Distinguishing sudden infant death syndrome from child abuse fatalities. *Pediatrics* 2001; **107**: 437–441.

27. Maternal and Child Health Research Consortium. *CESDI 7th Annual Report.* London: Maternal and Child Health Research Consortium, 2000; <www.cesdi.org.uk/publications>.

28. Centers for Disease Control and Prevention. *Guidelines for Death Scene Investigation of Sudden Unexplained Infant Deaths: Recommendations of the Interagency Panel on Sudden Infant Death Syndrome. MMWR* 1996; **45**: 1–22.

29. Bass M., Kavath RE, Glass L. Death-scene investigation in sudden infant death. *N Engl J Med* 1986; **315**: 100–105.

30. Fleming PJ, Blair PS. Sudden unexpected deaths after discharge from the NICU. *Semin Neonatol* 2003; **8**: 159–167.

Scott A. Halperin

3

Fatal pertussis

Pertussis (whooping cough) is a severe respiratory infection caused by *Bordetella pertussis*, a small, fastidious, slow-growing, Gram-negative coccobacillus. In the typical infection, upper respiratory symptoms of rhinorrhea and mild cough develop after an incubation period of 7–10 days. This first phase of symptoms (the catarrhal phase) is indistinguishable from the common cold. After another 7–14 days, the cough increases in frequency and severity and comes in fits, often worse at night. The change in the nature of the cough heralds the beginning of the paroxysmal phase which may last up to 4 weeks. During this phase, the cough is characterised by repetitive bursts of 5–10 coughs within the same expiration, with the patient often becoming red in the face and then cyanotic. During a coughing spasm, the child may have neck vein distension, bulging of the eyes, and tongue protrusion. The paroxysm may end with a whoop which is created as air is rapidly inspired against a closed epiglottis or end with vomiting and expulsion of a mucous plug. Paroxysms occur spontaneously but may also be precipitated by noise, eating or physical contact. Weight loss is common and can be significant. Complications may occur during this phase and include pneumonia, atelectasis, pneumothorax, retinal and conjunctival haemorrhage, hernia, seizures, and encephalopathy. Over time, the paroxysms become less severe and less frequent and the patient enters the convalescent phase which can last for several months. During this phase, the paroxysmal cough often recurs with any intercurrent viral respiratory infection. Although typical pertussis occurs in most children, manifestations of pertussis in infants, and adolescents and adults may vary. Young infants may present with apnoea and cyanosis and may never develop the typical cough or whoop. Adolescents and adults may simply present with prolonged cough and be misdiagnosed with bronchitis.

Scott A. Halperin MD
Professor of Pediatrics, Associate Professor of Microbiology & Immunology, Head, Pediatric Infectious Diseases, Director, Clinical Trials Research Center, Dalhousie University, IWK Health Centre, 5950/5980 University Avenue, Halifax, NS B3K 6R8 Canada
E-mail: scott.halperin@dal.ca

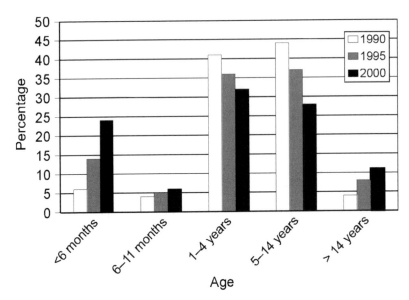

Fig. 1. Age distribution of pertussis in the UK in 1990, 1995, and 2000 following the gradual recovery of pertussis immunisation rates from a low of 20% in 1975 to the current levels of >95%.[46] The shift to higher incidence in infants under 6 months of age and a trend toward increased incidence in adolescents is notable.

Prior to widespread use of pertussis vaccine in the 1940s and 1950s, pertussis was a frequent cause of death in young children throughout Europe and North America. At present, the World Health Organization estimates that there are more than 300,000 deaths from pertussis each year, worldwide.[1] Although most of these deaths occur in the non-industrialised world where immunisation rates are low, deaths from pertussis continue to occur in young infants in industrialised nations that have achieved high rates of pertussis immunisation. This chapter will summarise the clinical, epidemiological and pathological features of severe pertussis and describe predictors of poor outcome.

EPIDEMIOLOGY

In the absence of universal pertussis immunisation programmes, pertussis is a frequent infection of pre-school-aged children, with over two-thirds of children having evidence of infection by 11–12 years of age.[2] With widespread use of vaccine, there is an early shift in peak incidence to infants under 1 year of age, with highest rates in infants too young to have completed the primary immunisation series (Fig. 1).[3] Recently, in countries with well-established pertussis vaccine programmes, there has been a further shift with a second peak in pre-adolescents and adolescents, likely a result of lapsed, vaccine-induced immunity.[4,5] An increasing number and proportion of cases are being reported in adults, raising the concern of transmission of pertussis by parents to very young infants.[6-9]

Deaths from pertussis have decreased dramatically since the widespread use of pertussis vaccine. Prior to universal pertussis immunisation, pertussis was amongst the leading killers of pre-school-aged children; in 1934, the year

Table 1 Incidence of fatal pertussis in selected industrialised nations with universal pertussis immunisation programmes

Country	Deaths	Deaths/100,000 population/ year[a]	Case fatality rate[a]	Estimate of under-reporting	Ref.
Australia	9 (1993–1997)	0.5	1/500[b]	–	46
Canada	16 (1991–2001)	0.36	1/111[b]	–	9, 11
UK	33 (1994–1999)	0.75	1/650	28%	16, 20
US	101 (1990–1999)	0.24	1/125–1/170	35%	12–14, 19

[a]Estimated, in children under 1 year of age.
[b]Estimated, in hospitalised children.

with a peak of just over 265,000 cases of pertussis recorded in the US, over 5000 deaths were reported.[10]

Deaths from pertussis have not been eliminated, even in countries with high rates of immunisation (Table 1). In Canada, 16 fatal cases of pertussis were reported to IMPACT, an active, hospital-based surveillance system that accounts for over 90% of the tertiary care paediatric hospital beds in the country.[11] In the US, 27,826 cases of pertussis were reported to the Centers for Disease Control (CDC) between 1980 and 1989 (average 2782 cases/year)[12] increasing to 29,134 cases between 1997 and 2000 (average 7283 cases/year).[13] In the 1980s, the CDC received reports of 77 deaths from pertussis (1.67 deaths per million) which increased to 103 deaths in the 1990s (2.4 deaths/million).[14] In New South Wales, Australia, 4 fatal cases were reported in one year from 1996 to 1997.[15] In England and Wales, 50 fatal cases were reported between 1980 and 1992, during a period when vaccine coverage rose from its low of under 33% in the mid-1970s to 91% by 1992.[16]

Although reporting of pertussis is suboptimal, cases in infants, hospitalised cases and fatal cases are reported with the highest frequency;[12,17,18] despite this, fatal cases of pertussis are still under-reported. In the US, using capture-recapture methodology that compares fatal cases reported to two independent surveillance systems, it was estimated that there was a total of 98 deaths from pertussis during the period (25 deaths/year) rather than the 32 and 23 cases reported to the two surveillance systems, respectively (underestimation of 35%).[18] For the 5-year period following this study, the estimate was an average of 31 deaths/year with 49% unreported to either surveillance system.[19] In a recent study using similar methodology in England and Wales, under-reporting was estimated at 28% (estimate of 46 cases rather than the 33 cases actually reported by the combination of the 3 data sources).[20] Misdiagnosis or failure to diagnose pertussis further adds to the under-reporting of fatal cases of pertussis. In Germany and the UK, analysis of deaths attributed to sudden infant death syndrome (SIDS) reveals that a proportion of these deaths are due to pertussis. In the UK, increases in SIDS incidence coincided with community outbreaks of pertussis.[21] In Germany, polymerase chain reaction analysis of SIDS deaths showed that 9 (18%) of 51 tested were in fact due to pertussis.[22] This decreased to 5.1% after widespread implementation in Germany of universal infant immunisation against pertussis.[23]

Most deaths from pertussis occur in young infants, particularly those too young to have completed their primary immunisation series. In Canada, of the 16 deaths reported to IMPACT, all occurred in infants 6 months of age or younger and 15 in infants younger than 2 months of age.[11] Only one infant who died had received a dose of pertussis vaccine (a 6-month-old who had only received a single dose). In the US, 20 (87%) of the 23 deaths reported in 1992–1993 were under a year of age; 18 (90%) were under 6 months and 11 (55%) were under 2 months of age.[24] More recently, the distribution of deaths has continued to shift toward the younger cohorts with all of the deaths reported in children under 4 months of age.[25] Similar results have been reported from England and Wales (83% of the deaths in infants under the age of 3 months)[26] and from Australia.[15] Despite the predominance of deaths in young infants, it should be noted that deaths from pertussis still occur in children over one year of age[16,24] and pertussis deaths have been reported in adults and in the elderly.[27]

PATHOLOGY AND PATHOGENESIS

Although the clinical manifestations of pertussis are well described, the pathogenesis of these signs and symptoms is incompletely understood. *B. pertussis* produces a wide array of toxins – including pertussis toxin, tracheal cytotoxin, adenylate cyclase toxin and an endotoxin (lipo-oligosaccharide) – that affect haematological and epithelial cell function. Although it is hypothesised that the actions of these toxins lead to the clinical manifestations, there is no definitive proof. For example, pertussis toxin is the most important of these toxins, produced only by *B. pertussis*. In mice, pertussis toxin produces lymphocytosis, sensitisation to the effects of histamine, hypoglycaemia as a result of activation of pancreatic islet cells, and inhibition of phagocytosis by monocytes and macrophages. Although it is attractive to hypothesise that pertussis toxin causes the paroxysmal cough and these other effects in human pertussis, they are also present in infections caused by *Bordetella parapertussis* which has the gene that encodes pertussis toxin but does not express it.[28]

Complications associated with pertussis are typically due to the results of the increased intrathoracic pressure related to the paroxysmal coughing; examples include pneumothorax, inguinal and umbilical hernias, conjunctival and retinal haemorrhages, and rib fractures and urinary incontinence in older children and adults. Airway mucous plugging can lead to atelectesis and secondary (non-pertussis) bacterial pneumonia. Central nervous system complications of seizures and encephalopathy may be the result of either hypoxic damage that occurs during paroxysmal coughing or from microhaemorrhages resulting from cough-related increased intracranial pressure.

Most of the deaths from pertussis in young infants are respiratory in nature, although central nervous system involvement is common. In the very young infant, there is typically diffuse involvement of the lungs with a primary bronchopneumonia and alveolar haemorrhage caused by *B. pertussis* (Fig. 2), although superinfection with other bacterial pathogens may occur just prior to death. There is a diffuse infiltration of acute and chronic inflammatory cells with both an interstitial and intra-alveolar distribution; organisms are easily

A

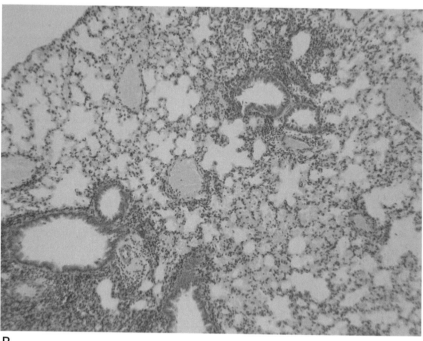

B

Fig. 2. Histopathology of the lung of (A) a 34-day-old child who died from pertussis and (B) a 21-day-old mouse infected with *B. pertussis*. Haematoxylin and eosin stained; magnification 10x objective plus digital zoom. The human lung pathology can be readily duplicated in the animal model by establishing a primary *B. pertussis* pneumonia. I thank Dr James Wright for the preparation of the histological specimens and photographs.

Table 2. Clinical characteristics of 16 fatal and 32 non-fatal cases of pertussis

Symptom/sign	Percentage with sign/symptom	
	Fatal cases	Non-fatal cases
Clinical presentation		
Cough	100	91
Cough with vomiting	56	55
Cough with cyanosis	63	75
Cough with paroxysms	56	87*
Whoop	0	19*
Apnoea	40	48
Complications		
Pneumonia	94	19*
Atelectasis	63	19*
Pneumothorax	6	0
Hernia	6	0
Seizures	21	0*
Hospital course		
Intensive care admission	100	37*
Intubation/ventilation	100	67*
Admission white blood cell count (per litre)	49.0×10^9	19.9×10^{9}*

Adapted from Mikelova et al.[11]
*$P < 0.05$.

identified with the inflammatory cells. Anoxic tissue damage is often seen in multiple organs including the brain, the heart, the liver (acute hepatic necrosis) and the kidney (acute tubular necrosis). Other organ damage can occur, although the pathophysiology is not certain.[29] Death from pertussis in older children is uncommon and postmortem studies are not usually available. Secondary bacterial pneumonia is more common, often with pathogens typically seen in hospital-acquired infection (*Pseudomonas aeruginosa* or *Klebsiella pneumonia*, for example).[30]

CLINICAL FEATURES AND PREDICTORS OF FATAL PERTUSSIS

Children with fatal pertussis segregate into two major groups according to clinical features of their disease: those that die early, likely as a result of unrecognised apnoea and bradycardia, and those who die as a result of pneumonia or another complication of their disease. Pertussis in young infants can present with apnoea without the presence of cough or other pertussis symptoms. If the apnoeic event is unobserved and unrecognised, death can occur; in these cases, a mis-diagnosis of SIDS may be made.[21–23] If recognised and brought to medical attention, the apnoea is typically managed and the infants usually develop other manifestations of pertussis illness. In these cases, the prognosis is more related to the extent of their respiratory involvement than to the apnoea. Early in the clinical course (at the time of presentation to medical attention), there is little to distinguish a case of pertussis that will lead to death from one that will recover (Table 2). In an analysis of 13 critically ill infants with pertussis, a white blood cell count $> 100 \times 10^9/l$ was a predictor of a fatal outcome.[31] In a case-control study of 16 fatal cases of pertussis,[11] only the white blood cell count predicted fatal cases from non-fatal cases at the time of hospital admission (73% of fatal cases and 86% of non-fatal cases); however, there was no specific white blood cell count that discriminated fatal from non-fatal cases. As the hospitalisation progressed and the child worsened, fatal cases were virtually always transferred to an intensive care unit. During hospitalisation, only white blood cell count was predictive of a fatal outcome (62% of fatal cases and 86% of non-fatal cases); at the time of intensive care unit transfer, only presence of pneumonia was predictive of a fatal outcome (94% of fatal cases and 83% of non-fatal cases). During the intensive care unit stay, fatal cases were marked by their clinical deterioration, with a higher proportion than non-fatal cases requiring intubation and ventilation, use of non-standard methods of ventilation and extracorporeal membrane oxygenation, and/or use of broad-spectrum antimicrobial agents.

MANAGEMENT

Management of typical cases of pertussis consists of administration of antibiotics (Table 3) and re-assurance of the patient and family that the cough and symptoms will eventually (but not rapidly) resolve. Antibiotics, unless given in the catarrhal or early paroxysmal stage, do not have a substantial effect on the clinical course although there may be some shortening of the period of whooping;[32] they are effective in eliminating the pathogen from the nasopharynx and thereby decreasing the likelihood of person-to-person transmission. Most clinical experience in treatment of pertussis has been with erythromycin which eradicates the organism within 5 days; 10–14-day courses have been recommended but 7 days has been shown to be as effective as 14

Table 3 Antimicrobial dosage guidelines for pertussis

Drug	Paediatric dose	Adult dose[a]	Duration	Ref.
Erythromycin[b]	40 mg/kg/day in three divided doses	1 g in three divided doses	7 days	33
Azithromycin	10 mg/kg/day once daily for 1 day followed by 5 mg/kg/day once daily for 4 days	500 mg once daily for 1 day followed by 250 mg once daily for 4 days	5 days	34
Clarithromycin	15 mg/kg/day in two divided doses	500 mg twice daily	7 days	35
Trimethoprim-sulfamethoxazole[c]	8 mg/kg/day of trimethoprim/ 40 mg/kg/day sulfamethoxazole in two divided doses	160 mg trimethoprim/ 800 mg sulfamethoxazole twice daily	14 days	

[a]And maximum paediatric dose.
[b]Erythromycin estolate is the preferred preparation.
[c]Use only in presence of macrolide allergy or resistance; little data on efficacy

days.[33] High rates of gastrointestinal complaints are associated with the use of erythromycin; newer macrolides (azithromycin[34] for 5 days and clarithromycin for 7 days[35]) have been shown to be equally effective and better tolerated. Although erythromycin resistance has been described, it has only rarely been associated with poor outcome.[36] Symptomatic relief has been advocated with cough medications, inhaled β-adrenergics and steroids; however, none of these interventions have demonstrated benefit.

In young infants with pertussis, the cornerstone of management is hospitalisation and close observation. Intensive care admission may be required for management of apnoea, for worsening respiratory status as a result of pneumonia, or rarely for management of intractable seizures. Tracheal intubation and mechanical ventilation may be required to manage apnoeic episodes or because of hypoxaemia; the latter is consistent with a more malignant course and poor outcome.[37] Rapid deterioration is often associated with the development of pulmonary hypertension that is typically not responsive to hyperventilation, alkalinisation, or vasodilators including phosphodiesterase-III inhibitors (e.g., amrinone, milrinone) or nitrous oxide.[30,31,38,39] Attempts to use non-traditional ventilatory methods such as high-frequency jet ventilation or oscillatory ventilation have not met with much success. More recently, extracorporeal membrane oxygenation has been used, also without much success. Three reviews of an extracorporeal membrane oxygenation registry based in Ann Arbor, Michigan, found 22 cases of extracorporeal membrane oxygenation for pertussis over the 11 years from 1986–1997,[40] an additional 13 cases between 1997 and 1999,[41] and another 26 cases up until July 2002.[42] The mortality rate was 70.5% which compared unfavourably with extracorporeal membrane oxygenation for other paediatric indications including all respiratory causes (14–35%), cardiac disease (45%) and all other causes (38.55%).[42] Recently, it has been hypothesised that the pulmonary hypertension may be due to the high lymphocyte numbers and leukocyte adhesins with subsequent vascular obstruction and that improvement might be obtained through their reduction;[43] however, there are no data to support this and no recommendation can be made. Given the small number of cases that occur in the industrialised world, a therapeutic trial would need to be based on all tertiary care centres working together to evaluate treatment modalities.

Given the logistical difficulties of multicentre trials, focusing on preventing disease in young infants through neonatal or maternal immunisation may be the more practical route. With acellular pertussis vaccine, some efficacy has been demonstrated after one or two doses in the primary series;[44] protection against fatal pertussis may be provided even after the first dose. Pertussis vaccination can be given as early as 6 weeks; there are no data yet available on the use of a birth dose as is done with hepatitis B vaccine. Although there are data demonstrating decreased antibody levels later in infancy in neonates immunised with tetanus/diphtheria and whole cell pertussis vaccines,[45] there is no evidence that this occurs with acellular pertussis vaccine. The immunisation of women immediately after delivery has been proposed in order to provide a 'protective cocoon' around the newborn infant, although the effectiveness of this strategy has not been tested. Maternal immunisation has been proposed to provide transplacental antibodies, although whether placentally derived antibodies provide protection is controversial. Historically, when maternal protection was the result of naturally acquired infection, the immediate postnatal period was one of relative, although short-lived, protection. There is little evidence that there is much protection provided to the newborn from mothers whose immunity is largely (waned) vaccine-induced immunity. It is not known whether this is a result of differences in the nature of the immune response after infection or immunisation or a quantitative difference in the residual immunity retained by the mother. Further studies are required to understand better the nature of the immune response and protection of the newborn infant.

Key points for clinical practice

- The epidemiology of pertussis is changing with a shift of the peak incidence to young infants under 6 months of age and to adolescents and adults.

  The highest incidence is in infants too young to have completed the primary immunisation series.

  A second peak is in adolescents and adults, likely the result of waning immunity from the last dose of pertussis vaccine given in early childhood.

  Young infants acquire pertussis from older siblings and parents. Pertussis should be suspected in older children and adults with a prolonged, non-improving cough.

- Deaths from pertussis continue to occur in well-immunised populations in industrialised nations.

- Prevention through immunisation is the most effective strategy but current practice still leaves the youngest infants vulnerable.

  On-time commencement of the infant immunisation schedule is of utmost importance given that perhaps the first and certainly the second dose of the primary series provide some protection.

  Chemoprophylaxis with a macrolide antibiotic is generally recommended for infant contacts of cases of pertussis.

- Pertussis in young infants may have an atypical presentation; a high index of suspicion is required so that the diagnosis is not missed. Pertussis can be severe in young infants; most deaths occur in infants who have not received any doses of pertussis vaccine.

  An infant with new onset of apnoea should be evaluated for pertussis.

  Pertussis should be considered in any infant with a cough illness who is a close contact of a child, adolescent or adult with prolonged cough illness.

  Infant deaths from pertussis may be misdiagnosed as SIDS. Proper specimens should be obtained at postmortem examination to rule out pertussis.

  Young infants with pertussis should be observed in hospital, with highest priority given to those who have not yet started their immunisation series. *continued on next page continued from previous page*

- **Management of pertussis includes antimicrobials and dose monitoring for evidence of apnoea, and respiratory compromise.**

  Erythromycin, clarithromycin and azithromycin are all effective in eradicating *Bordetella pertussis* from the nasopharynx. The latter two are associated with fewer side effects.

  Antimicrobials prevent further transmission of the organism but do not substantially modify the clinical course.

  Antitussive agents, β-adrenergics and inhaled steroids have not been shown to be effective in relieving the symptoms of pertussis.

  High white blood cell counts are correlated with more severe disease. Bronchopneumonia is associated with a more severe outcome. Onset of pulmonary hypertension is highly associated with a fatal outcome.

  Extracorporeal membrane oxygenation has not been an effective modality of management of the pulmonary complications of pertussis.

References

1. World Health Organization. *Facts and Figures. The World Health Report 2003 – Shaping the future.* <http://www.who.int/whr/2003/en/Facts_and_Figures-en.pdf> Accessed 16 July, 2004.
2. Stroffolini T, Giammanco A, De Crescenzo L *et al*. Prevalence of pertussis IgG antibodies in children in Palermo, Italy. *Infection* 1989; **17**: 280–283.
3. Tanaka M, Vitek CR, Pascual FB, Bisgard KM, Tate JE, Murphy TV. Trends in pertussis among infants in the United States, 1980–1999. *JAMA* 2003; **290**: 2968–2975.
4. Yih WK, Lett SM, des Vignes FN, Garrison KM, Sipe PL, Marchant CD. The increasing incidence of pertussis in Massachusetts adolescents and adults, 1989–1998. *J Infect Dis* 2000; **182**: 1409–1416.
5. Skowronski DM, De Serres G, MacDonald D *et al*. The changing age and seasonal profile of pertussis in Canada. *J Infect Dis* 2002; **185**: 1448–1453.
6. Beiter A, Lewis K, Pineda EF, Cherry DJ. Unrecognized maternal peripartum pertussis with subsequent fatal neonatal pertussis. *Obstet Gynecol* 1993; **82**: 691–693.
7. Smith C, Vyas H. Early infantile pertussis; increasingly prevalent and potentially fatal. *Eur J Pediatr* 2000; **159**: 898–900.
8. Hoppe JE. Neonatal pertussis. *Pediatr Infect Dis J* 2000; **19**: 244–247.
9. Halperin SA, Wang EEL, Law B *et al*. Epidemiological features of pertussis in hospitalized patients in Canada, 1991–1997: Report of the Immunization Monitoring Program – Active (IMPACT). *Clin Infect Dis* 1999; **28**: 1238–1243.
10. Centers for Disease Control. Annual summary 1982: reported morbidity and mortality in the United States. *MMWR Morb Mortal Wkly Rep* 1983; **31**(54): 59–61, 147.
11. Mikelova LK, Halperin SA, Scheifele D *et al*, members of the Immunization Monitoring Program, Active (IMPACT). Predictors of death in infants hospitalized with pertussis: A case control study of 16 pertussis deaths in Canada. *J Pediatr* 2003; **143**: 576–581.
12. Farizo KM, Cochi SL, Zell ER, Brink EW, Wassilak SG, Patriarca PA. Epidemiological features of pertussis in the United States, 1980–1989. *Clin Infect Dis* 1992; **14**: 708–719.
13. Centers for Disease Control and Prevention. Pertussis – United States, 1997–2000. *MMWR Morb Mortal Wkly Rep* 2002; **51**: 73–76.
14. Vitek CR, Pascual RB, Baughman AL, Murphy TV. Increase in deaths from pertussis among young infants in the United States in the 1990s. *Pediatr Infect Dis J* 2003; **22**: 628–634.
15. Williams GD, Matthews NT, Choong RKC, Ferson MJ. Infant pertussis deaths in New South Wales 1996–1997. *Med J Aust* 1998; **168**: 281–283.

16. Miller E, Vurdien JE, White JM. The epidemiology of pertussis in England and Wales. *Commun Dis Rep CDR Rev* 1992; **2**: R152–R154.
17. Halperin SA, Bortolussi R, MacLean D, Chisholm N. Persistence of pertussis in an immunized population: Results of the Nova Scotia Enhanced Pertussis Surveillance Program. *J Pediatr* 1989; **115**: 686–693.
18. Sutter RW, Cochi SL. Pertussis hospitalizations and mortality in the United States, 1985–1988: Evaluation of the completeness of national reporting. *JAMA* 1992; **267**: 386–391.
19. Shaikh R, Guris D, Strebel PM, Wharton M. Underreporting of pertussis deaths in the United States: Need for improved surveillance [letter to the editor]. *Pediatrics* 1998; **101**: 323.
20. Crowcroft NS, Andrews N, Rooney C, Brisson M, Miller E. Deaths from pertussis are underestimated in England. *Arch Dis Child* 2002; **86**: 336–338.
21. Nicoll A, Gardner A. Whooping cough and unrecognized perinatal mortality. *Arch Dis Child* 1988; **63**: 41–47.
22. Heininger U, Stehr K, Schmidt-Schläpfer G et al. *Bordetella pertussis* infections and sudden unexpected deaths in children. *Eur J Pediatr* 1996; **155**: 551–553.
23. Heininger U, Kleemann WJ, Cherry JD and the Sudden Infant Death Syndrome Study Group. A controlled study of the relationship between *Bordetella pertussis* infections and sudden infant deaths among German infants. *Pediatrics* 2004; **114**: e9–e15. URL: <http://www.pediatrics.org/cgi/content/full/114/1/e9>.
24. Wortis N, Strebel PM, Wharton M, Bardenheier B, Hardy IRB. Pertussis deaths: Report of 23 cases in the United States, 1992 and 1993. *Pediatrics* 1996; **97**: 607–612.
25. Centers for Disease Control and Prevention. Pertussis deaths – United States, 2000. *MMWR Morb Mortal Wkly Rep* 2002; **51**: 616–618.
26. Ranganathan S, Tasker R, Booy R, Habibi P, Nadel S, Britto J. Pertussis is increasing in unimmunised infants: is a change in policy needed? *Arch Dis Child* 1999; **80**: 297–299.
27. Centers for Disease Control and Prevention. Fatal case of unsuspected pertussis diagnosed from a blood culture – Minnesota, 2003. *MMWR Morb Mortal Wkly Rep* 2004; **53**: 131–132.
28. Hausman SZ, Cherry JD, Heininger U, Wirsing von König CH, Burns DL. Analysis of proteins encoded by the *ptx* and *ptl* genes of *Bordetella bronchiseptica* and *Bordetella parapertussis*. *Infect Immun* 1996; **64**: 4020–4026.
29. Hackman R, Perrin DG, Karmali M, Cutz E. Fatal *Bordetella pertussis* infection: Report of two cases with novel pathologic findings. *Pediatr Pathol Lab Med* 1996; **16**: 643–653.
30. Gillis J, Grattan-Smith T, Kilham H. Artificial ventilation in severe pertussis. *Arch Dis Child* 1988; **63**: 364–367.
31. Pierce C, Klein N, Peters M. Is leukocytosis a predictor of mortality in severe pertussis infection? *Intensive Care Med* 2000; **26**: 1512–1514.
32. Bergquist SO, Bernander S, Dahnsjo H, Sundelof B. Erythromycin in the treatment of pertussis: a study of bacteriologic and clinical effects [published erratum appears in *Pediatr Infect Dis J* 1987;6:1035]. *Pediatr Infect Dis J* 1987; **6**: 458–461.
33. Halperin SA, Bortolussi R, Langley JM, Miller B, Eastwood BJ. Seven days of erythromycin estolate is as effective as fourteen days for the treatment of *Bordetella pertussis* infections. *Pediatrics* 1997; **100**: 65–71.
34. Langley JM, Halperin SA, Boucher FD, Smith B; Pediatric Investigators Collaborative Network on Infections in Canada (PICNIC). Azithromycin is as effective and better tolerated than erythromycin estolate for the treatment of pertussis. *Pediatrics* 2004; **114**: e96–e101. URL: <http://pediatrics.aappublications.org/cgi/content/full/114/1/e96>.
35. Lebel MH, Mehra S. Efficacy and safety of clarithromycin versus erythromycin for the treatment of pertussis: a prospective, randomized, single blind trial. *Pediatr Infect Dis J* 2001; **20**: 1149–1154.
36. Lee B. Progressive respiratory distress in an infant treated for presumed pertussis [Your Diagnosis, Please]. *Pediatr Infect Dis J* 2000; **19**: 475, 492–493.
37. Pilorget H, Montbrun A, Attali T et al. La coqueluche maligne du petit nourisson [Malignant pertussis in the young infant]. *Arch Pediatr* 2003; **10**: 787–790.
38. Goulin GD, Kaya KM, Bradley JS. Severe pulmonary hypertension associated with shock and death in infants infected with *Bordetella pertussis* [Case reports]. *Crit Care Med* 1993; **21**: 1791–1794.

39. Casano P, Pons Odena M, Cambra FJ, Martín JM, Palomeque A. *Bordetella pertussis* infection causing pulmonary hypertension [letter]. *Arch Dis Child* 2002; **86**: 453–454.
40. Williams GD, Numa A, Sokol J, Tobias V, Duffy BJ. ECLS in pertussis: does it have a role? *Intensive Care Med* 1998; **24**: 1089–1092.
41. Sreenan CD, Osiovich H. Neonatal pertussis requiring extracorporeal membrane oxygenation [Case report]. *Pediatr Surg Int* 2001; **17**: 201–203.
42. Halasa NB, Barr FE, Johnson JE, Edwards KM. Fatal pulmonary hypertension associated with pertussis in infants: Does extracorporeal membrane oxygenation have a role? *Pediatrics* 2003; **112**: 1274–1278.
43. Peters MJ, Pierce CM, Klein NJ. Mechanisms of pulmonary hypertension in *Bordetella pertussis* [letter]. *Arch Dis Child* 2003; **88**: 92–93.
44. Olin P, Rasmussen F, Gustafsson L, Hallander HO, Heijbel H. Randomised controlled trial of two-component, three-component, and five-component acellular pertussis vaccines compared with whole-cell pertussis vaccine. Ad Hoc Group for the Study of Pertussis Vaccines [published erratum appears in *Lancet* 1998;**351**:454]. *Lancet* 1997; **350**: 1569–1577.
45. Van Savage J, Decker MD, Edwards KM, Sell SH, Karzon DT. Natural history of pertussis antibody in the infant and effect on vaccine response. *J Infect Dis* 1990; **161**: 487–492.
46. Kirkbride H, White J. Chapter 5, Infectious Diseases. In: *The Health of Children and Young People* [online]. UK: Office for National Statistics; 2004: 1–31. <http://www.statistics.gov.uk/Children/ downloads/infec_disease.pdf>.

Jason Barling Jonathan Hourihane

4

Latex allergy

Latex allergy exists in the paediatric population and other high-risk groups, and the main aim in its management should be to prevent its development. To understand this problem fully, it is necessary to look at the origins of natural rubber latex and in what ways patients and staff are exposed to it. This chapter considers the routes of sensitisation, reaction severity, and methods of diagnosis.

NATURAL RUBBER LATEX

Natural rubber latex is an aqueous elastomer emulsion originating from about 2000 plant species. It is composed mainly of water (55–65%) and rubber (30–40%), with the next main component being protein (2.3%). It is formed in the cytoplasm of cells called 'laticifers' which form a tube-like network in plants and function to seal damaged sites. The process by which the rubber particles form is complex and is thought to involve a protein, hevein, around which the particles aggregate and an enzyme, rubber elongation factor (Hev b1), that is involved in formation of the rubber chain. Whilst the proteins that are involved in natural rubber synthesis are most likely to be found only in natural rubber latex, the laticifer cells also contain plant defence enzymes that are found in natural rubber latex as well as other fruits and vegetables

Jason Barling MBBS BSc MRCPCH
Paediatric SpR, Allergy & Inflammation Division, Welcome Trust Clinical Research Facility, Mailpoint 218, Southampton General Hospital, Tremona Road, Southampton SO16 6YD, UK
E-mail: BamboJase@aol.com (for correspondence)

Jonathan Hourihane MB DM MRCPI FRCPCH
Senior Lecturer, Division of Infection Inflammation and Repair, Welcome Trust Clinical Research Facility, Mailpoint 218, Southampton General Hospital, Tremona Road, Southampton SO16 6YD, UK
E-mail: j.hourihane@soton.ac.uk

(chitinases, glucanases). These proteins are thought to form the basis behind the origins of latex allergy and give a potential route to accurate diagnosis and treatment.

Latex has only been commercially available from the *Hevea brasiliensis* rubber tree, which is mainly grown in SE Asia and West Africa. The trees are cut at the base to allow collection of the latex, a process which has more recently been increased by hormone treatment and selective breeding. About 90% of production goes into 'dry natural rubber goods' (*e.g.* tyres, shoes, cables) where it is often combined with synthetic rubber. Dry rubber manufacturing involves a coagulation process which reduces the protein content. The remaining 10% produces 'latex concentrate' in which the tapped latex is stabilised with ammonia and then centrifuged. The concentrate is then prepared for dipping by a complex chemical process known as 'compounding'. The latex proteins are released into the concentrate during processing and may well be denatured but may also reveal a group of chemical- and heat-resistant proteins. Most concentrate is now used for dipped latex goods which include many medical and household items.

HISTORY

Latex was used as early as 1600 BC where it has been identified in balls used in games. It was not until the process of vulcanisation, a process of stabilisation by adding sulphur and improving the elasticity and thermostability, that it was possible to form a rubber glove; surgical gloves have been regularly used since 1900.[1] The use of rubber gloves has dramatically reduced the incidence of postoperative infections and became standard practice in the early 1900s.

The first recorded reaction to natural rubber was in 1927 following exposure to rubber in dental treatment. However, it was not until 1979 that the first immediate-type allergic reaction was reported in a housewife wearing a pair of rubber gloves.[2] By 1984, the first report of anaphylaxis to surgical gloves was described in two women undergoing obstetric and gynaecological procedures.[3]

There are several theories behind the apparent increase in the incidence of latex allergy.[1] One possibility is the increased use of latex gloves associated with the advent of AIDS and the adoption of 'universal precautions' in both medicine and everyday life. It will be difficult to determine whether this increased use increased sensitisation, symptoms or the rate of recognition of latex allergy. Another theory is that it may reflect the change in practice of using cornstarch to powder gloves. This has now been shown to act as an allergenic carrier promoting sensitisation. More controversially, it could be because the chemicals now used to enhance or stabilise yields promote allergenicity, but there are no convincing studies to endorse this theory. Finally, it is likely that there has been a greater awareness among the allergy communities and the general public and, therefore, a greater pick-up rate (so-called bias of ascertainment). The amount of research published, at least 1400 papers, over the past 20 years would certainly support this, compared to no papers being found on a Medline search between 1900–1984. To confound this issue even further, the accurate diagnosis of true latex allergy has been fraught with difficulty and it may be that we are just over diagnosing the condition, possibly confusing sensitisation and clinical allergy.

PATHOPHYSIOLOGY

The main risk groups for latex allergy are healthcare workers, patients with a history of multiple operations, and patients with co-existing allergies.

By 1983, the IgE-mediated pathogenesis of natural rubber latex allergy was confirmed and subsequently 200 allergens have been identified, with the major ones listed in Table 1. These allergens differ with respect to their source material and the patient group studied. This has been exemplified when comparing allergens in the two major risk groups – healthcare workers and patients with congenital abnormalities. Healthcare workers recognise more water-soluble proteins such as Hev b5 and Hev 6.02, whereas spina bifida patients react to more hydrophobic proteins, *e.g.* Hev b1 and Hev 3. This may reflect the fact that healthcare workers are exposed through inhalation or wearing latex gloves whereas spina bifida patients undergo multiple operations and have to use in-dwelling catheters repeatedly. It is also supported by the fact that children who have not undergone any surgical procedures have a pattern that resembles the healthcare workers.[4]

CROSS-ALLERGIES

Latex-fruit syndrome

When looking at those with latex sensitisation, it has been shown that about 50% have allergies to foods.[5] The foods identified most frequently include potato, avocado, banana, tomato, chestnut and kiwi. Studies have also looked at children with co-existing allergies and found 1–2% of this group are sensitised to latex, often without a history of unusual exposure.[6]

As there does not seem to be a botanical basis for this observation, the question of cross-reactivity of specific IgE-binding proteins was raised. This has led to the name 'latex-fruit syndrome'. Serological inhibition tests have demonstrated cross-reacting IgE antibodies between natural rubber latex and allergens in other plants. This can be explained by peptide homology between

Table 1 Some allergens identified in natural rubber latex

Systematic name	Conventional name	Function	Affected subject groups
Hev b1	Rubber elongation factor	Biosynthesis of polyisoprene chain	80% spina bifida 50% healthcare workers
Hev b3	Rubber particle protein	Rubber synthesis and latex coagulation	80% spina bifida 20% healthcare workers
Hev b5	Acidic C-serum protein	Structural protein	92% healthcare workers, 56% spina bifida
Hev b6	Prohevein		
Hev b6.01	Hevein		80% healthcare workers
Hev b6.02	Prohevein C-domain	Latex coagulation	30% spina bifida

rubber latex and other plant proteins. With further development of diagnostic tests for latex and other allergies, the proteins causing specific allergy have been identified. Three types of hydrolytic enzymes – glucanases, chitinases and acidic esterases – have been identified from IgE antibodies of patients with latex allergy. These enzymes are involved in plant protection against infection and attack. Antibodies to these enzymes have also been identified in patients with allergies to various foods.[7]

It is no surprise, therefore, that almost half of latex-sensitised patients also display an associated fruit allergy.[8] What is more uncertain, however, is whether patients develop sensitivity to fruit through latex exposure or the other way around.

ROUTE OF EXPOSURE

More than 40,000 medical and household products are made from latex but the quoted prevalence of latex allergy in the general population is fortunately less than 1%.[9] Allergens may cause sensitisation through multiple routes, including cutaneous, mucosal and parenteral, but impact on the skin and mucous membranes appears to provide the main source of exposure. Natural rubber latex gloves and catheters are responsible for the majority of immediate-type reactions in healthcare settings. This may be from occupational exposure, examination, barium enema, obstetric procedures and surgery.[10] However, exposure may also occur during leisure activities[10] or during protected intercourse.[11] Appropriate advice needs to be given to latex-allergic teenagers regarding barrier methods of contraception.

Whilst in the adult population of healthcare workers, epidemiological studies have shown correlation between general latex glove use and allergy,[12] it has been harder to show an exposure–response relationship because of difficulty in classifying outcomes. Exposure studies have identified that powdered gloves increase the airborne allergen levels,[13] but this may be confounded by the fact that gloves with a higher protein concentration produce more airborne allergen. There have also been supporting studies showing a reduction in latex-specific IgE found in hospitals where powder-free gloves are used.[14,36]

When looking at a population that has undergone multiple operations, children with spina bifida show the highest prevalence of natural rubber latex sensitisation. They are especially at risk because of the combination of early and repeated surgery as well as congenital urological abnormalities. Within the paediatric population, there is growing evidence to link the number of operations with risk of latex allergy.[15] One UK study has shown that having had a single previous operation increases the odds of latex sensitisation 13-fold.[8] More recent evidence in children with chronic renal failure has analysed the operations separately and shown that only urological surgery was significantly associated with latex reaction.[16] Not surprisingly, therefore, it has also been shown that establishing a latex-free operating theatre for these patients has been very successful in primary prevention.[17]

Co-existing atopy is the most important predisposing factor for natural rubber latex sensitisation. The presence of atopy may increase the risk of sensitisation between 4.4–25-fold.[18]

It has been suggested that exposure to latex at birth provides the stimulus for later allergy and that premature babies are at great risk, but there are no data to support this suggestion. Studies have also looked at children receiving home ventilation and found a significant proportion of them that were sensitised to latex.[19] It is not known, however, whether they were sensitised prior to, or during, the use of ventilation.

SENSITISATION

There remains much confusion about terminology in allergy, 'Sensitisation' is defined as the presence of a positive skin prick test or specific IgE antibody in serum to a particular antigen. The term sensitisation does not automatically equate with clinical reactivity or 'allergy' which describes the physical, often immediate, symptoms that are produced when a sensitised individual is exposed. 'Hypersensitivity', on the other hand, is often a delayed response not associated with IgE antibodies.

When looking at sensitisation to other allergens, certain principles have been noticed.[6]

ALLERGEN EXPOSURE IS A RISK FACTOR FOR IGE SENSITISATION AND AN EXPOSURE–RESPONSE RELATIONSHIP EXISTS

Comparing the incidence of latex sensitisation in the general population 0.8–6.5%[20] with those who are regularly exposed where it is as high as 72%,[21] it is apparent that latex exposure is a risk factor to sensitisation. When looking at surgical exposure in children, seroconversion can occur after 2% of repeat operations in an unselected group.[8] This is confirmed in children with spina bifida where in longitudinal studies we see evidence of an exposure–response relationship, with increasing levels of latex antibody following exposure in surgery.[22]

CO-EXISTING ATOPY STEEPENS THE EXPOSURE–RESPONSE RELATIONSHIP

In all populations, the prevalence of latex allergy has been associated with atopy. Within the paediatric age group, there has been shown to be a significant association between latex sensitisation and the presence of one or more positive skin prick test responses to aero-allergens, food allergens, or both; one or more positive skin prick test responses to one or more insect venoms; and older age. It was also noticed that latex sensitisation was only present in atopic children.[23]

SENSITISATION USUALLY OCCURS A FEW YEARS AFTER INITIAL EXPOSURE

Although it is sometimes difficult to identify the time of initial exposure, sensitisation is thought to occur a few years later. The subsequent time to onset of symptoms and, therefore, allergy has then varied from less than 3 months to more than 20 years. This probably reflects the large variation in amount of allergen and route of exposure to which people respond. It also makes it difficult in further defining the exposure–response relationship when it is hard to quantify the level of exposure.

REACTION SEVERITY

As with most allergy, the severity of reaction varies hugely between individuals. It can range from mild contact urticaria, through local airway compromise to anaphylactic shock (Table 2). The difficulty is not judging where the patient is along this gradient, but predicting where they might end up. Studies that have looked into factors that influence the presence of symptoms have shown that the main risk factor in sensitised children is the number of operations and that co-existing atopy both lower the threshold for sensitisation and for clinical reactions.[24] This problem is further confounded by the fact that latex products also vary hugely in their protein composition and subsequent allergenic potential. Latex producers have tried to help with this problem by stating the latex content, but this is not universal. It has also been suggested that individuals may have a genetic susceptibility that determines the degree of antibody production to a particular allergen and this may influence the reaction severity.[25]

As most non-operative exposure to latex of healthcare workers occurs via the skin, one might expect the most frequent reaction to be cutaneous. This does not seem to be the case, as upper and lower respiratory symptoms are more frequent than cutaneous symptoms.[26] This may reflect the fact that, as in the case of healthcare workers, there is both cutaneous and airborne allergen involved in sensitisation. The possibility also exists that respiratory symptoms are more likely to be reported and the connection made between exposure and symptoms.

Obviously, the most serious concern is anaphylaxis during surgery the incidence of which is between 1:5000 to 1:25,000 with a mortality of 3.4%.[27] Latex is now the second most common cause of anaphylaxis during surgery.[28] When looking at latex-sensitive children in a high-risk group, 30% presented with anaphylaxis.[29] It may be suspected by the fact that it often occurs during maintenance anaesthesia with a delay of 30–60 min, as opposed to during induction when muscle relaxants – the most common cause of intra-operative anaphylaxis – are given intravenously. Latex anaphylaxis has, however, also been reported following other medical interventions such as barium enemas and dental procedures. Attempts have been made to develop pre-operative

Table 2 Reaction severity in different organs

Cutaneous	Pruritis
	Erythema
	Urticaria
	Angioedema
Eyes	Conjunctivitis
	Angioedema
Nasal	Rhinitis
Bronchial	Stridor
	Bronchospasm
Gastrointestinal	Abdominal cramping
	Nausea/vomiting
Cardiac	Tachycardia
	Hypotension
	Death

questionnaires in order to assess the risk of latex sensitivity so that testing can be performed and appropriate measures taken.[28] Such questionnaires seem a sensible idea, but have not been validated or universally adopted as yet.

DIAGNOSIS

Investigation of all allergy relies primarily on a good history followed by the combination of using pure, standardised allergens to perform skin prick testing with the assessment of specific IgE antibody response. The gold standard investigation is then finally a controlled exposure to the specific allergen within a safe environment. However, as discussed later, skin prick test solutions and specific IgE tests are not yet standardised. When applying this to latex allergy, the diagnostic algorithm illustrated in Figure 1 may be helpful:

CLINICAL HISTORY

When taking a clinical history, the main aim is to assess the risk group for the child. This may be done by dividing the assessment into: (i) medical history, *e.g.* presence of atopy and history of anaphylaxis during procedures; and (ii) surgical history, *e.g.* multiple operations and unexplained peri-operative events.

Despite a thorough history, not all latex-sensitive patients will be identified and a number of false-positive histories will be recorded. It is, therefore, important to use appropriate investigations to confirm or exclude the diagnosis.

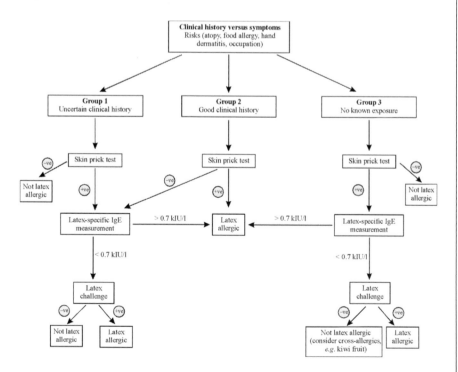

Fig. 1 Algorithm for determining latex allergy response.

TEST RELIABILITY

When developing the diagnostic tests for latex allergy, it was found that latex contains a large number of proteins and that there is variation in content between batches. At least 10 allergenic proteins have now been classified, but it may be that only a combination of a few are required to confirm the diagnosis.[30] As previously described, a further problem with these proteins is the cross-reactivity they display with other allergens, *e.g.* banana, grass pollen, *etc.* The difficulty is, therefore, in interpreting the results with any degree of certainty and reproducibility. One possible solution to this might be the use of recombinant proteins, which would also provide a standardised method of diagnosis.[30] These approaches have not reached the paediatric clinic yet.

Skin prick test

Skin prick tests have been performed with latex glove extracts for some time, but the difficulty has been to create a standardised preparation. Comparison of extracts has concluded that non-ammoniated latex was the most practical and reproducible reagent.

When looking at diagnostic accuracy, studies have also quoted a sensitivity of 93–96% and specificity of 96–100% when using non-ammoniated latex for intradermal and puncture skin tests.[31] They have also concluded that such tests are inherently safe when the protein concentration is monitored.[31] A level of 100 mcg/ml of non-ammoniated latex has been found to be a safe concentration, but dilutions of 1 and 10 mcg/ml should used if there is a strong history of severe reaction. It is important to recognise that such accuracy is dependent on a good clinical history and an approved standardised reagent. Intradermal tests are not recommended and normal epicutaneous procedures should be used.

Latex-specific IgE

Serological testing has not been as reliable as skin prick tests as there is considerable difference in reactivity of IgE antibody with different antigens.[32] The first commercial *in vitro* assay was approved by the US Federal Drug Administration in 1995 and, subsequently, further assays have been released. When their performance is compared, diagnostic sensitivity is between 75–100% and specificity between 67–97%.[33] Further studies have also shown that such assays are imprecise when antibody levels are near the positive cut-off value (0.35–0.45 kIU/l) and that duplicate tests should be performed.[34] Ideally, IgE antibodies to purified allergens could improve the accuracy but, as yet, these are not commercially available.

Latex challenge

In vivo controlled exposure to an allergen provides the most effective determination of the patient's allergic status. The main difficulty with respect to latex is providing a standardised way of exposure, with a known allergy content, that can also be masked from the patient. Different approaches have been tried from inhalation of aqueous surgical glove extract[35] to provocation with glove wearing and sequential glove inflation.[36] Provocation tests tend to be reserved for patients with a conflicting history and initial investigations as

Table 3 Glove provocation test

> Natural rubber latex challenge undertaken on children's day ward according to protocol. Child must remain on ward for minimum of 2 h following challenge whatever the result. Antihistamine therapy must be stopped prior to challenge
>
> Challenge should not be performed if child has any open/weeping eczematous areas on the hand. This could induce a severe anaphylactic reaction, due to increased absorption of allergen
>
> An anaphylaxis kit, resuscitation facilities and medical staff must be available
>
> Latex-free gloves must be worn by staff handling the test substance to avoid cross contamination and so that hand contact does not start a further reaction in the child

there is always a small risk of anaphylaxis. To ensure safety, there must be a quantifiable allergen exposure and an objective end point to determine outcome. It is technically possible to quantify exposure in an inhalational test using a hood or chamber, but these are not routinely available. It must be done in a centre experienced in performing exposure challenges so that appropriate safety measures are taken. Table 3 depicts the challenge scheme used in our centre.

REGIMEN

Stage 1
Latex glove on left hand and latex-free glove on right hand for 5 min and then observe for 15 min.

Stage 2
Place both hands in water and repeat stage 1.

Stage 3
Repeat stage 2 for 30 min and observe for 2 h.

Discharge advise
The child should rest for the remainder of the day as activity may induce a delayed reaction. If the challenge is positive then advice is needed regarding exposure avoidance and Epipen training. Accurate documentation is required in the medical notes in case of further admissions and medic alert and support leaflets given.

HOPE FOR TREATMENT

PRIMARY PREVENTION

It appears that latex allergy originates from a combination of the intensity of latex exposure, route of sensitisation and genetic susceptibility. One could, therefore, logically conclude that by reducing the exposure one might reduce the incidence of allergy. It may also be said that by being aware of this potential problem in childhood and identifying those at greatest risk, a strong argument could be put forward for minimising early and recurrent exposure to latex of those identified as high-risk for latex sensitisation. One study to support this has been carried out in Germany where a change to latex-free gloves has been linked with a reduced number of cases of latex-induced bronchial hyper-reactivity.[37] The same group has looked at contact urticaria caused by latex in healthcare workers and concluded that a reduced number of proven cases are associated with a reduced purchase of powdered gloves.[38] A 'before and after study' has also suggested that primary prevention may reduce the incidence of latex sensitisation in children with spina bifida.[39] Further research is required to confirm the cost-effectiveness of this approach.

The practical way in which prevention is implemented also needs to be considered. For example: (i) education of those at risk about natural rubber latex allergy and methods of exposure; and (ii) introduction of latex-free environments and, if latex gloves are to be used, use powder-free products to reduce allergenicity.

The difficulties associated with this are: (i) quantification of the allergen in materials is easier said than done, despite some attempts at labelling; (ii) latex allergens are present in many other products, including cross-reactivity with certain fruits and vegetables (it is difficult to avoid them all); (iii) some latex-free products do not satisfy the requirements of normal use made on them as well as their latex counterparts (*e.g.* surgical gloves); and (iv) most latex-free products are significantly more expensive but this must be balanced against the loss of workforce and compensation of healthcare workers and the future medical costs for patients, that may be required after latex sensitisation.

DISEASE MANAGEMENT (SECONDARY PREVENTION)

Once diagnosed with natural rubber latex sensitisation or actual latex allergy, the most important goals are first to avoid further exposure and second to be aware of the management of symptoms caused by accidental exposure.

Exposure avoidance

If patients with latex allergy come into hospital, it must be into a latex-free environment. All latex-allergic patients should have a medic alert bracelet and staff must be made aware of the risks of exposure.

If surgery is anticipated then there needs to be an established protocol on how to manage latex allergy safely. The patient should be first on the day's list to avoid contamination. Currently, there is no evidence that pretreatment with antihistamines or corticosteroid confers any protection against anaphylaxis.[40]

Patients also need to be aware of alternatives to non-medical rubber products such as condoms and the risk of possible reactions to fruits.

Symptom management

As always, the difficulty comes in predicting those patients who have a less severe reaction but who will get worse with further exposure. It is important, therefore, to describe the risks of exposure, especially in healthcare environments. Medical exposure can usually be predicted and severe reactions outside clinical care settings are unusual. There remains a risk for those who need home care and those who have already had significant reactions not related to medical care. Asthma appears to be a strong risk factor for anaphylaxis outside the hospital, irrespective of the implicated allergen. The importance of asthma needs to be considered carefully in decisions about Epipens.

POSSIBLE CURE

In the absence of standardised allergens, it is difficult to predict if treatments such as desensitisation and immunotherapy can be developed. With the occurrence of anaphylaxis during skin-prick tests, the main concern with classical immunotherapy is the risk of adverse events. A trial evaluating safety and clinical efficacy after 6 months of subcutaneous immunotherapy has shown benefit on cutaneous symptoms. However, 8% of doses induced systemic reactions mainly during the build-up phase.[41] Sublingual desensitisation has been suggested as an alternative route with less risk of reactions. Initial studies have shown some improvement in symptoms when assessed 3 months after a 4-day regimen with no side effects.[42] Not surprisingly, none of these studies have been performed in children and it may be some time yet before this is a possibility.

At present, whilst work on recombinant allergens looks promising, management will remain focused on prediction of exposure and hopefully wide-spread adoption of prevention strategies.

Key points for clinical practice

- Unless we look for latex allergy, it will find us, and probably find us unprepared.

- The main risk groups for latex allergy are healthcare workers, patients with a history of multiple operations, and patients with other allergies.

- A significant proportion (about half) of those with latex allergy have associated allergies to other foods.

- Natural rubber latex gloves and catheters are responsible for the majority of immediate-type reactions in healthcare settings.

- The main risk factors for presence of symptoms in sensitised children is the number of operations and co-existing atopy; both lower the threshold for sensitisation and for clinical reactions.

- Latex is now the second most common cause of anaphylaxis during surgery.

- Diagnosis of latex allergy depends on a good clinical history and appropriate use of investigations.

- Baseline investigations should involve standardised solutions for skin prick tests and measurement of specific IgE.

(continued on next page)

(continued from previous page)

- The gold standard test for diagnosing latex allergy is an exposure challenge which must be carried out in an experienced unit with strict protocols.

- Primary prevention is currently the main hope for latex allergy. This will require education of those at risk and providing evidence of the cost-benefit of its implementation.

- Management of existing latex allergy requires increased understanding of those at risk of sensitisation and management protocols to avoid further exposure.

References

1. Ownby D. A history of latex allergy. *J Allergy Clin Immunol* 2002; **110**: S27–S32.
2. Nutter F. Contact urticaria to rubber. *Br J Dermatol* 1979; **101**: 597–598.
3. Turjanmaa K. Severe IgE mediated allergy to surgical gloves (abstract). *Allergy* 1984; **39**: S2.
4. Yitalo L, Alenius H, Turjanmaa K, Palosuo T, Reunala T. IgE antibodies to prohevein, hevein and rubber elongation factor in children with latex allergy. *J Allergy Clin Immunol* 1998; **102**: 659–664.
5. Beezhold DH, Sussman GL, Liss GM, Chang NS. Latex allergy can induce clinical reaction to specific foods. *Clin Exp Allergy* 1996; **26**: 416–422.
6. Weissman D, Lewis D. Allergic and latex specific sensitization: route, frequency and amount that are required to initiate IgE production. *J Allergy Clin Immunol* 2002; **110**: S57–S63.
7. Yamagi T, Sato T, Nakamura A *et al*. Plant-defense-related enzymes as latex allergens. *J Allergy Clin Immunol* 1998; **101**: 379–385.
8. Cullinan P, Brown R, Field A *et al*. Latex allergy. A position paper of the British Society of Allergy and Clinical Immunology. *Clin Exp Allergy* 2003; **33**: 1484–1499.
9. Turjanmaa K, Makinen-Kiljunen S, Reunala T *et al*. Natural rubber latex allergy – the European experience. *Immunol Allergy Clin North Am* 1995; **15**: 71–88.
10. Axelsson IGK, Eriksson M. IgE-mediated anaphylactoid reactions to rubber. *Allergy* 1987; **42**: 46–50.
11. Levy DA, Khonader S. Allergy to latex condoms. *Allergy* 1998; **53**: 1107–1108.
12. Slater JE. Latex allergy. *J Allergy Clin Immunol* 1994; **94**: 139–149.
13. Heilman DK, Jones RT, Swanson MC, Yunginger JW. A prospective study showing that rubber gloves are the major contributor to latex aeroallergen levels in the operating room. *J Allergy Clin Immunol* 1996; **98**: 325–330.
14. Allmers H, Brehler R, Chen Z *et al*. Reduction of latex aeroallergens and latex specific IgE antibodies in sensitised workers after removal of powdered natural rubber latex gloves in a hospital. *J Allergy Clin Immunol* 1998; **102**: 841–846.
15. Hourihane J, Allard J, Wade A, McEwan A, Strobel S. Impact of repeated surgical procedures on the incidence and prevalence of latex allergy: a prospective study of 1263 children. *J Pediatr* 2002; **140**: 479–482.
16. Sparta G, Kemper M, Gerber AC, Goetschel P, Neuhaus TJ. Latex allergy in children with urological malformation and chronic renal failure. *J Urol* 2004; **171**: 1647–1649.
17. Cremer R, Kleine-Diepenbruck U, Hoppe A, Blaker F. Latex allergy in spina bifida patients – prevention by primary prophylaxis. *Allergy* 1998; **53**: 709–711.
18. Moneret-Vautrin DA, Beaudouin E, Widmer S *et al*. Prospective study of risk factors in natural rubber latex hypersensitivity. *J Allergy Clin Immunol* 1993; **92**: 668–677.
19. Nakamura C, Ferdman R, Keens T, Ward S. Latex allergy in children on home mechanical ventilation. *Chest* 2000; **118**: 1000–1003.
20. Anon. AORN latex guideline. *Association of Operating Room Nurses Journal* 1999; 93–108.

21. Ricci G, Gentili A, DiLorenzo F et al. Latex allergy in subjects who had undergone multiple surgical procedures for bladder exstrophy: relationship with clinical intervention and atopic diseases. *BJU Int* 1999; **84**: 1058–1063.

22. Cremer R, Hoppe A, Kleine-Diepenbruck U, Blaker F. Longitudinal study on latex sensitisation in children with spina bifida. *Pediatr Allergy Immunol* 1998; **9**: 40–43.

23. Bernardini R, Novembre E, Ingargiola A et al. Prevalence and risk factors of latex sensitisation in an unselected pediatric population. *J Allergy Clin Immunol* 1998; **101**: 621–625.

24. Mazon A, Nieto A, Estornell F et al. Factors that influence the presence of symptoms caused by latex allergy in children with spina bifida. *J Allergy Clin Immunol* 1997; **99**: 600–604.

25. Rihs HP, Chen Z, Rueff F et al. HLA-DQ8 and the HLA-DQ8-DR4 haplotype are positively associated with the hevein-specific IgE immune response in health care workers with latex allergy. *J Allergy Clin Immunol* 2002; **110**: 507–514.

26. Ho A, Chan H, Tse KS et al. Occupational asthma due to latex in health care workers. *Thorax* 1996; **51**: 1280–1282.

27. Fisher MM, More DG. Epidemiology and clinical features of anaphylactic reactions in anaesthesia. *Anaesth Int Care* 1981; **9**: 226–234.

28. Lieberman P. Anaphylactic reactions during surgical and medical procedures. *J Allergy Clin Immunol* 2002; **110**: S64–S69.

29. Kwittken PL, Sweinberg SK, Campbell DE, Pawlowski NA. Latex hypersensitivity in children: clinical presentation and detection of latex specific IgE. *Pediatrics* 1995; **95**: 693–699.

30. Sussman G, Beezhold D, Kurup V. Allergens and natural rubber proteins. *J Allergy Clin Immunol* 2002; **110**: S33–S39.

31. Hamilton RG, Adkinson Jr NF. Natural rubber latex diagnostic skin testing reagents: safety and efficacy of non-ammoniated latex, ammoniated latex and latex rubber glove extracts. *J Allergy Clin Immunol* 1996; **98**: 872–873.

32. Kurup VP, Kelly KJ, Turjanmaa K et al. Immunoglobulin E reactivity to latex antigens in sera of patients from Finland and the US. *J Allergy Clin Immunol* 1993; **91**: 1128–1134.

33. Hamilton RG, Peterson EL, Ownby D. Clinical and laboratory-based methods in the diagnosis of natural rubber latex allergy. *J Allergy Clin Immunol* 2002; **110**: S47–S56.

34. Biagini R. Receiver operating characteristics and reproducibility analyses of FDA cleared latex specific IgE assays (abstract). *J Allergy Clin Immunol* 2000; **106**: S82.

35. Marias C, Lazaro M, Fraj J et al. Occupational asthma due to latex surgical gloves. *Ann Allergy* 1991; **67**: 319–323.

36. Niggeman B, Buck D, Michael T, Wahn U. Latex provocation tests in patients with spina bifida: who is at risk of becoming symptomatic? *J Allergy Clin Immunol* 1998; **102**: 665–670.

37. Allmers H, Schmengler J, Skudlik C. Primary prevention of natural rubber latex allergy in German health care system through education and intervention. *J Allergy Clin Immunol* 2002; **110**: 318–323.

38. Allmers H, Schmengler J, John SM. Decreasing incidence of occupational contact urticaria caused by natural rubber latex allergy in German health care workers. *J Allergy Clin Immunol* 2004; **114**: 347–351.

39. Nieto A, Mazon A, Pamies R et al. Efficacy of latex avoidance for primary prevention of latex sensitisation in children with spina bifida. *J Pediatr* 2002; **140**: 370–372.

40. Setlock MA, Cotter TP, Rosner D. Latex allergy: failure of prophylaxis to prevent severe reactions. *Anesth Analg* 1993; **76**: 650–657.

41. Sastre J, Fernandez-Nieto M, Rico P et al. Specific immunotherapy with a standardized latex extract in allergic workers: a double-blind placebo-controlled study. *J Allergy Clin Immunol* 2003; **111**: 985–994.

42. Patriarca G, Nucera E, Pollastrini E et al. Sublingual desensitisation: a new approach to latex allergy problem. *Anesth Analg* 2002; **95**: 956–960.

L. Gareth Evans-Jones Rolfe Birch

5

Congenital brachial palsy

We review the current state of knowledge in this potentially disabling condition and refer to new work in risk factors, natural history, definition of prognosis, operative repair of the nerve and recognition of shoulder dislocation. We hope to assist the clinician to select the infant that requires specialist assessment and, if appropriate, surgical treatment.

TERMINOLOGY AND DEFINITION

The terminology is confusing – obstetrical brachial plexus palsy, brachial plexus neuropathy, Erb's palsy and congenital brachial palsy (CBP) are all terms in current use. We prefer the latter as it has no implications on the aetiology and the term commonly used by paediatricians, Erb's palsy is a variety of CBP, albeit the commonest. CBP can be defined as a flaccid paresis of an arm, rarely both arms, presenting at birth when on examination, the range of passive motion of the arm is greater than the active.[1,2]

CLASSIFICATION

The most useful classification is that first described by Narakas based on clinical findings in the first weeks of life:[3]

    Group I   Paralysis of shoulder and biceps (C5 & C6).

L. Gareth Evans-Jones MBBS MRCP FRCPCH (for correspondence)
Consultant Paediatrician, Countess of Chester Hospital NHS Foundation Trust, Liverpool Road, Chester CH2 1UL, UK
E-mail gareth.evans-jones@coch.nhs.uk

Rolfe Birch Mchir FRCS, FRCS(Eng by election)
Professor of Orthopaedic Neurological Surgery, Peripheral Nerve Injury Unit, Royal National Orthopaedic Hospital NHS Trust, Brockley Hill, Stanmore, Middlesex HA7 4LP, UK

Group II   Paralysis of shoulder, biceps and forearm extensors (C5, C6 & C7). Groups I and II constitute Erb's palsy with Group II cases differing from Group I because of wrist extensor involvement.

Group III   Complete paralysis of the limb (flail arm) – (C5–TI)

Group IV   As in III with ipsilateral Horner syndrome due to sympathetic chain involvement.

Injury to C8 and T1 roots alone causing a claw hand – Klumpke's paralysis, described in association with breech delivery, is rare.[4,5] In the first national survey of the incidence, risk factors and natural history of CBP in the British Isles (conducted under the auspices of the British Paediatric Surveillance Unit), Evans-Jones and co-workers found no cases of Klumpke's paralysis.[6] Of the cases studied, 91% were in Groups I and II and 6.5% in Groups III and IV compared with other studies where the proportion of cases in Groups I and II varied from 42% to 87%.[1,2] They also reported the right arm to be more commonly affected than the left (50% versus 43%) with five bilateral cases. The incidence of bilateral lesions has been reported to be 20% of cases following breech delivery.[4]

INCIDENCE

Up until recently, the incidence of CBP in the British Isles was unknown.[1,2]. In the British Paediatric Surveillance Unit survey of 776,618 infants born in the UK and Republic of Ireland in 1998–1999 there were 323 confirmed cases giving an incidence of 0.42 per 1000 (1 in 2300) although the authors state that their study may underestimate the incidence by up to 11%.[6] Adler and Patterson in New York reported a reduction in the incidence of CBP from 1.56 per 1000 in 1938 to 0.38 per 1000 in 1962, strikingly similar to that of the British Paediatric Surveillance Unit survey and ascribed the reduction to improved obstetric care.[7] It is postulated that the incidence may have increased in recent years because of the trend of increasing birth weight despite improved obstetric care, increased caesarean section rates, decreased vaginal breech deliveries, better identification and management of shoulder dystocia and other factors.[1,2,6]

PATHOGENESIS AND RISK FACTORS

CBP is a lesion of the brachial plexus (or part of it) but there has been much controversy as to whether injury occurs before or at delivery. It is traditionally held that CBP is the result of excessive traction at birth. There are three well documented risk factors – the heavy baby, shoulder dystocia and breech delivery. Shoulder dystocia is one of the most unpredictable and frightening obstetric emergencies with a significant mortality and morbidity including CBP. In the past 10 years, guidelines have been produced leading to regularly practised drills in most obstetric departments.[8] There is, however, no evidence that appropriate management of shoulder dystocia leads to a reduction in the incidence of CBP.[9] In a study of over a million births in Sweden between 1987 and 1996, Christofferson and Rydhystrom reported an incidence of 1.3 cases of shoulder dystocia per 1000 live births of which 26% had CBP.[10] Clements reported that CBP has overtaken cerebral palsy as a subject of litigation for the obstetrician.[11]

Jennet and colleagues reported an incidence of 56% of 'unexplained cases' in a retrospective study of 57,597 births from 1977 to 1990 in which only 39 cases were identified.[12] The authors compared the characteristics of 17 of infants whose delivery was complicated by shoulder dystocia and 22 infants without shoulder dystocia. Although the latter group included infants delivered by assisted delivery, breech extraction, caesarean section, and prolonged second stage of labour they proposed the cause as 'intra-uterine maladaptation'. Later reports proposed that CBP is not always the result of excessive traction to the brachial plexus with lateral flexion of the head by the obstetrician or midwife in order to deliver the anterior shoulder impacted on the symphysis pubis. Gherman and co-workers suggested that a significant number of cases of CBP followed *in utero* trauma, and reported CBP in the posterior arm of infants whose deliveries were complicated by shoulder dystocia of the anterior shoulder.[13] The brachial plexus is also not immune from injury at caesarean section particularly if the infant is large or very preterm.[14]

Gonik and colleagues described a mathematical model to estimate the compressive pressure on the fetal neck overlying the roots of the brachial plexus by the symphysis pubis during shoulder dystocia.[15] They compared the estimated compressive pressure from clinician-applied traction (exogenous forces) and the estimated uterine and maternal expulsive efforts (endogenous forces) and demonstrated that the latter were > 4 times greater than the former suggesting that, in a significant number of cases, endogenous *in utero* pressure on the brachial plexus may be the cause of injury. Increasingly, other authors subscribe to this 'maternal propulsive theory' and we also find the hypothesis persuasive.

Evans-Jones *et al.*[6] found shoulder dystocia was associated with 60% of infants with CBP, high birth weight with 53%, and assisted delivery 36% – all of these features were significant. Compared with the general population, significantly fewer infants with CBP were delivered by caesarean section. Breech delivery was reported in only 3% of cases probably reflecting the reduction in vaginal breech deliveries in the UK (1% in England, 1994–1995).[16] Other injuries were noted in 15% of cases (Table 1). In 29 (9%) of the reported

Table 1 Associated injuries[6]

Bony injuries		26 (8%)
	Fracture of clavicle	11
	Fracture of humerus	8
	Shoulder dislocation	7
Other nerve injuries		9 (3%)
	Horner's syndrome	5
	Facial palsy	3
	Phrenic nerve palsy	1
Soft tissue injuries		12 (4%)
	Facial and other bruising	8
	Cephalohaematoma	3
	Sternomastoid tumour	1

cases, there were no clear indications of the occurrence of unusual force in the course of the delivery but other factors were identified in 10 babies – there were two concealed pregnancies with delivery at home, three deliveries after prolonged labour, three delivered by emergency LSCS including one hand presentation, one normal delivery in a mother with a history of previous shoulder dystocia and one following successful external cephalic version for breech presentation (previously unreported). Thus the true incidence of unexplained cases was probably lower than 9%.

Injury to the brachial plexus varies in extent and severity although, in general, the more extensive the injury the more severe it is. The uppermost roots and trunks are the most vulnerable to injury. There are four types of nerve injury that may occur (Fig. 1):

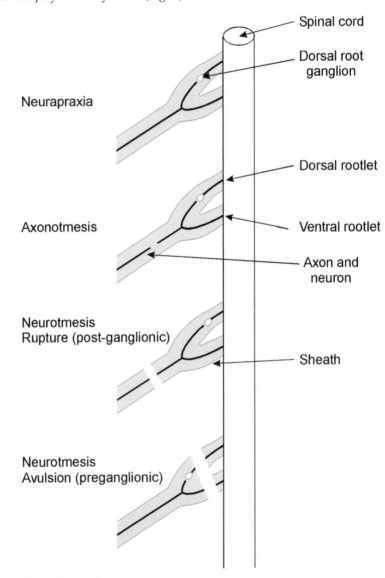

Fig. 1 Types of nerve injury.

1. **Neurapraxia** where the myelin sheath only is damaged producing a conduction block which is reversible.

2. **Axonotmesis** where there is disruption of some or all of the axons but preservation of the sheath allowing recovery.

3. In **neurotmesis** there is (i) rupture (postganglionic) or (ii), in the worst case, the spinal nerve is torn from the spinal cord – a preganglionic, avulsion, injury. A high incidence of this injury affecting the upper nerves is seen in breech CBP.[4,5]

The difficulties in assessing the degree and extent of the injury at presentation and early infancy is at the heart of the debate on the place and timing of surgery.

DIAGNOSIS AND ASSESSMENT

Diagnosis is usually straightforward with a newborn infant showing lack of active movement of an arm but with full passive motion at the shoulder, elbow and wrist joints on gentle examination. The most important differential diagnosis is injury to the shoulder, clavicle, humerus, or forearm when passive motion is restricted by pain and muscle spasm. External signs of bony and other injuries should be sought and only when the examiner is happy that bony injuries are not present should a detailed full examination be performed of the central nervous system including primitive and peripheral reflexes in all four limbs aiming in particular to exclude cervical cord injury.[1] An ipsilateral Horner syndrome should be actively sought. In an infant with respiratory difficulty presenting at birth, a chest radiograph should be obtained to exclude phrenic nerve (C3–C5) palsy, a particular complication of breech CBP lesions.[4,5] Observation of the infant's spontaneous movements and posture is often the most useful part of the assessment, with in cases in Groups I and II, for example, the infant adopting the classical 'waiter's tip' posture with preservation of the function of the small muscles of the hand (Fig. 2). Signs of muscle wasting, contracture and hypoplasia of the affected limb suggest a prenatal cause and in the British Paediatric Surveillance Unit survey one such case was described, possibly an asymmetrical variant of arthrogryposis or congenital cervical spinal muscular atrophy.[17]

In severe cases of CBP, there may be autonomic changes in the skin of the affected limb – coolness, dryness to the touch, and a marble like appearance. Insensitivity to pain and touch may be elicited in the affected dermatomes.

Table 2 Differential diagnosis

Bony injuries	May co-exist with CBP
Infection	Osteomyelitis of the humerus
	Osteomyelitis cervical spine with paraspinal abscess
Tumours	Myofibromatosis
	Haemangiomatosis
Cervical cord injury	
Arthrogryposis or congenital spinal muscular atrophy	
Familial	Autosomal dominant?
Iatrogenic	Complication of CPAP with Gregory box

Table 2 summarises other possible causes of unilateral monoparesis in the newborn infant.

ROLE OF OTHER INVESTIGATIONS

The place of radiological imaging in the assessment of CBP is uncertain. CT myelography is useful in identifying the presence of pseudomeningocoeles

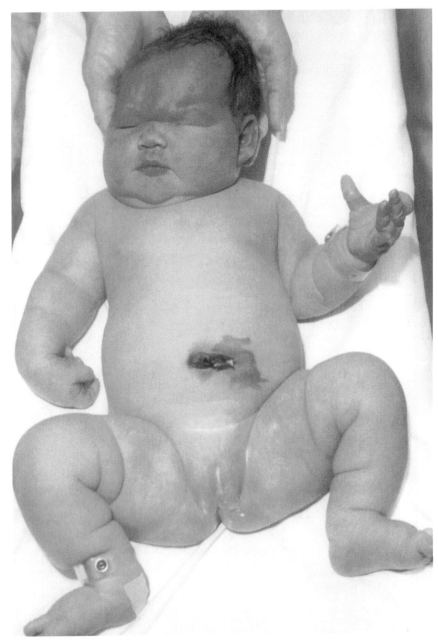

Fig. 2 A right Group II CBP in a newborn infant (birth weight 5 kg) of a diabetic mother showing a classical 'waiter's tip' posture.

associated with root avulsion and is more sensitive than advanced sequence MRI but is more invasive.[4,5] MRI, on occasion, can demonstrate neuromas associated with root rupture. With increasing experience, we believe that MRI will become the most useful imaging modality in selected cases, particularly when intraspinal avulsion injury is suspected.

Electromyography and nerve conduction velocities have, up until recently, been of limited usefulness, but there have been significant developments in this area which will be referred to later. They must be performed, and interpreted, by experts. They are seen as an adjunct to clinical examination. They are difficult to interpret within the first weeks of life and tend to be unduly pessimistic if performed within the first 10 weeks. At this stage of course, the examiner is recording physiological events for nerves which are still recovering; some nerve fibres have undergone a process of regeneration and are only at the early stages of spontaneous regeneration.

NATURAL HISTORY AND OUTCOME

The outcome in CBP is dependent on the extent and severity of the lesion with, in general, a better outcome in upper plexus than in lower or total plexus injuries.[18,19] The reported incidence of complete recovery, however, is very variable reflecting differences in the number and selection of populations studied, functional methods of assessment, definitions of degrees of recovery and age at assessment. In the British Paediatric Surveillance Unit survey of 276 cases evaluated at a median age of 23 weeks, 52% had recovered fully, 46% partially and 2% showed no recovery.[6] The risk of a poor outcome was significantly correlated with the extent of the injury with no Group III or IV cases out of 19 making a full recovery, with 68% making a partial recovery and 32% making no recovery – the comparative figures for Group I and II cases being 56%, 44% and 0% respectively, i.e. all Group I and II cases showed some useful recovery by 6 months of age. There was no significant increased risk of a poor outcome associated with high birth weight, assisted delivery or shoulder dystocia. The progression of recovery is centripetal, proceeding proximally so that shoulder abduction (C5) shows incomplete recovery more frequently than elbow extension (C7), for example 87% versus 39% out of 127 cases with partial recovery (Fig. 3). In summary, 73% of all cases studied had fully recovered elbow flexion at around 6 months of age.

There is ample evidence that if significant recovery is to occur at all, its rate of progression is relatively rapid in the first 3 months and then slows down. Bennett and Harrold reporting 24 cases noted that in those who fully recovered

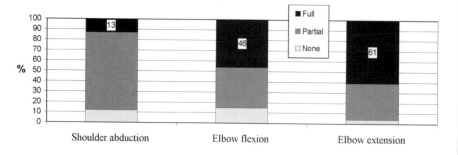

Fig. 3 Pattern of recovery at 6 months of age in 127 partially recovered infants.[6]

this was apparent by 5 months and early signs of recovery were seen within 2 weeks.[19] In a large series, Narakas pointed out that signs of recovery for C5 and C6 within 3 months was encouraging and that early return of finger flexion in total lesions was followed by good hand function.[3] Gilbert and colleagues in an influential work concluded that absence of biceps and deltoid contraction by 3 months of age was an accurate predictor of a poor outcome.[20] Michelow and co-workers devised a grading system to evaluate active movement of shoulder, elbow, wrist, thumb and finger muscles against gravity converting the measurements to a total numerical score in 66 infants with CBP at 3, 6, 9 and 12 months of age and found that although elbow flexion at 3 months was a useful predictor of a good outcome at 12 months, there was a false positive rate of 12.8% but when combined with elbow, wrist, thumb and finger extension in a total score this figure was reduced to 5.2%.[21] Other reported poor prognostic factors are an ipsilateral Horner syndrome, possibly phrenic nerve palsy and associated bony injuries.[22]

LONG-TERM OUTCOMES AND COMPLICATIONS

CBP is a potentially severely disabling condition. Severe extensive lesions (Groups III and IV) can cause a permanent flail and insensate arm.[23] This category is, fortunately, a small minority; however, even if some recovery occurs, the child can still be left with significant permanent disability – not only from the direct effects of nerve injury, but also from long-term complications due primarily to muscle contracture if not prevented.

The most common and the most serious of these secondary deformities is posterior subluxation – dislocation of the shoulder. This deformity requires treatment by operation in just under one-third of all cases of CBP.[24] The untreated case, in early adult life, presents a sorry picture of painful loss of function at the shoulder, abnormal posture of the upper limb as a whole, and a considerable impairment of elbow and of hand function. Untreated posterior dislocation of the shoulder is more crippling than untreated developmental dislocation of the hip.

Other common contractures affecting the shoulder include those involving the inferior muscles and soft tissues which diminish movement between the scapula and the humerus. In the more severe cases, the shoulder functions as an ankylosis. These deformities are particular common in Groups II and III and may reflect imperfect regeneration of the nerves with defects in the afferent pathway and, possibly co-contraction between antagonistic muscles. Such shoulder deformities interfere with the posture of the limb, and many parents will relate that their child falls over more frequently and that there is obvious deformity when the child is running.

Flexion deformity of the elbow is common, and causes apparent shortening of the arm.

In some of the more severe injuries to the brachial plexus, recovery of the 7th cervical nerve is particularly poor and these children demonstrate a supination posture of the forearm, with the wrist held in ulnar deviation, thumb in palm, and weakness of wrist extension.

Dislocation of the head of radius is uncommon. It is associated with more severe injuries involving C7 and C8 and it may lead to a secondary abnormality at the wrist joint.[25]

Sjoberg and colleagues, examining 11 cases of incompletely recovered CBP at 3–11 years of age, noted hypoplasia in the affected arm in every case which was more marked in the more extensive lesions.[26] Sensation was impaired in the hand in the two cases of flail arm studied with one exhibiting self-mutilation. The difficulties these children demonstrated were in activities such as eating, carrying a tray, dressing, adjusting shoulder straps, and playing a musical instrument.

MANAGEMENT

The aims of treatment can be summarised as: (i) achievement of maximal nerve injury recovery; (ii) maintenance of optimal passive ranges of movement and suppleness of affected joints; and (iii) strengthening of affected muscles. Addressing these aims provides the opportunity to minimise disability in the long term and requires the input of a multidisciplinary team of experts with a core team of specialist brachial plexus and orthopaedic surgeon, physiotherapist, occupational therapist, orthotist and paediatric anaesthetist. The services of a social worker and clinical psychologist may also be required and the local community paediatrician has a pivotal role to play.

INITIAL MANAGEMENT

This is usually the responsibility of the general paediatrician and physiotherapist with midwife support and is firstly conservative. The parents will need careful counselling and the wise paediatrician will review the diagnosis carefully in the first days of life, assess the severity and extent of the lesion and resist the temptation of inappropriately optimistic prognostication. In the first week, the arm should be rested and protected from excessive movement with physiotherapy withheld until the second week of life. The parents are instructed to treat the child at least three times a day – passively abducting and externally rotating the shoulder, placing the hands above the head, externally rotating the shoulder with the elbow flexed and kept at the infant's side and placing the back of the hand on the bed. These exercises should be performed with both arms simultaneously to stabilise the trunk and scapula.[18] To stretch the posterior scapulohumeral angle, the arm is stretched across the chest towards the other shoulder. The hand should also be placed behind the back and behind the head. The elbow, wrist and fingers should be put through all movements to prevent contractures. The best therapists are parents: the role of the physiotherapist is to teach, support, monitor and record progress (Fig. 4).

Figure 5 summarises the recommended referral pathway from the non-specialist centre to the specialist.

SURGERY

Nerve repair

The place and timing of nerve repair surgery has been well reported by Birch,[18] Gilbert,[20,25] and others.[1,2] Surgeons first operated on cases of CBP in the early part of the 20th century but surgery fell out of favour in the 1920s and 1930s and a more conservative approach was adopted until the advent of new microsurgical techniques in the 1980s. Experience was largely obtained in young men with traumatic brachial plexus lesions after, in particular, motor cycle accidents. The dilemma is in the selection of infants who will benefit from surgery and when to intervene. Studies of nerve injury and regeneration have

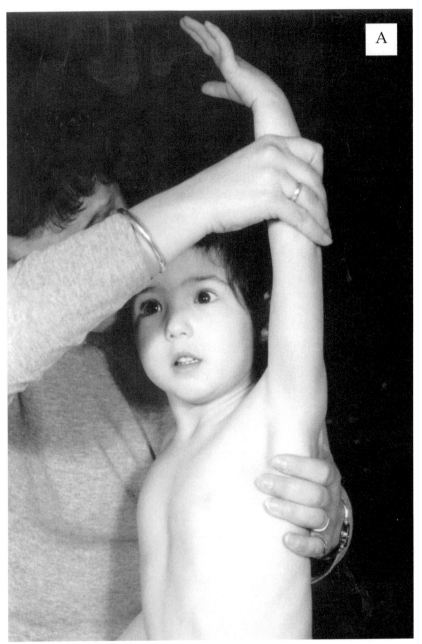

Fig. 4 A mother giving physiotherapy to her 3-year-old daughter with a Group II lesion causing marked stiffness and impending subluxation of the shoulder.
(A) Demonstrates the method of overcoming inferior contracture – note how the mother holds the scapula against the chest wall whilst fully elevating the arm.

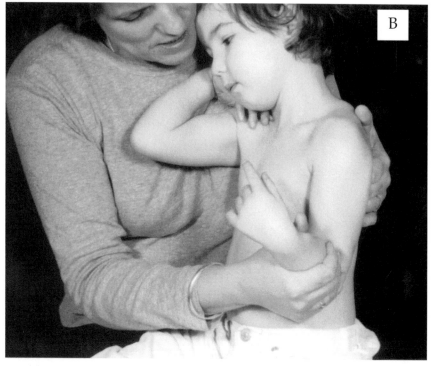

Fig. 4 (B) Demonstrates the technique for maintaining full lateral rotation of the shoulder – note how the arm is held in adduction, one hand stabilising the scapula whilst the other, gently but firmly rotates the arm laterally.

shown that the rate of recovery and final outcome of an injured nerve depends on the severity of the lesion so that in neurapraxia complete recovery can be expected in 3–4 months whilst in axonotmesis it may take many months; after rupture or avulsion the chance of significant spontaneous recovery is poor in the former, and nil in the latter which is not amenable to direct repair.[18,20,23]

Nerve injuries in children heal better than in adults and the nerves are shorter so that regeneration is more rapid. On the other hand, denervated muscle is believed to undergo irreversible loss of its neuromotor endplates after 12–15 months.[23] Thus there exists a window of opportunity for those children in whom surgery should be beneficial and specialist surgeons are increasingly of the view that surgical exploration is required within the first 6 months of life. The strongest advocates of this approach are Gilbert and colleagues based on extensive experience and data leading to the recommendation that if there is incomplete recovery of biceps at 3 months, surgical intervention is indicated.[25,27] Michelow and colleagues developed a muscle grading and scoring system of 10 different muscle actions at shoulder, elbow, wrist and fingers; these extended the work of Gilbert and colleagues to refine the accuracy of clinical assessment in predicting final outcome and are probably the best tools currently available.[21] However, Waters in a series of 66 patients confirmed Gilbert's observation that infants with no evidence of biceps function at 3 months rarely have complete recovery and that nerve repair improved the outcome in this small subgroup.[28] The problem, however,

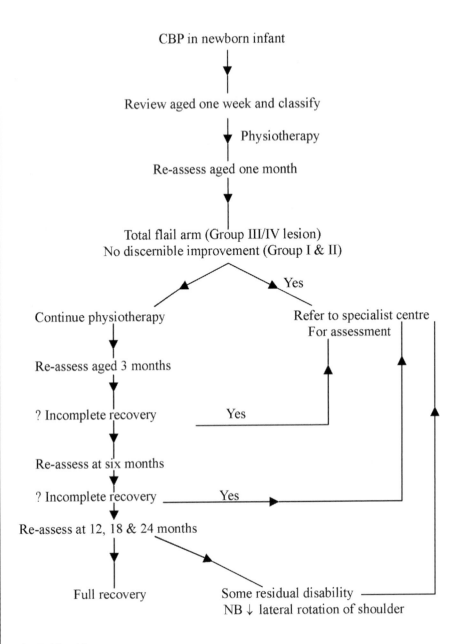

Fig. 5 Algorithm.

remains – how best to identify those who would benefit from surgery and the lack of hard evidence that the outcome would be improved in comparison to spontaneous recovery.

Clinical progress, or the lack of it, is the most important guide to long-term prognosis. Smith developed a system of neurophysiological examination in which compound nerve action potentials are recorded for median and ulnar nerves in the forearm and these are supplemented by electromyelographic examination of selected muscles in each myotome; deltoid for C5; biceps for

C6; forearm extensors for C7; forearm flexors for C8 and first dorsal interosseous for T1.[29] On the basis of these findings, Smith graded nerve lesion into types A, B, and C. Type B is sub-divided into favourable and unfavourable groups. Type A is consistent with prolonged conduction block, whilst type C indicates a deep axonopathy consistent either with rupture of the nerve or even avulsion.

Bisinella and co-workers analysed progress in 75 babies with slow recovery for C5, C6 and C7 lesions.[30] In many centres, they would have been subjected to operation. A remarkably high match between the neurophysiological prediction and the final functional outcome was shown for C6 and for C7. In the 5th cervical nerve, the neurophysiological prediction was a less reliable indication for final function recovery and they demonstrated that posterior dislocation was statistically a highly significant explanation for the failure of some of these nerve lesions to recover to the expected level.

Smith's work goes some way towards defining the indications for operation in seemingly unfavourable cases. If we take as an example the 6th cervical nerve, the neurophysiological pattern A or B favourable is consistent with complete recovery of elbow flexion and forearm supination. Lesion B unfavourable is consistent with useful recovery of elbow flexion but limited range in power and imperfect supination. Lesion C is consistent with failure of recovery of elbow flexion. The 7th cervical nerve lesion A and B favourable is consistent with full recovery of finger and wrist extension. In B unfavourable, it is likely that there will be defects of wrist extension and in type C lesions it is highly unlikely that useful spontaneous recovery of wrist extension will occur. For the 5th cervical nerve, the type A lesion is consistent with full function of the shoulder. B favourable, on the other hand, predicts useful but incomplete recovery, with abduction or forward flexion of the shoulder of the order of 90–100°. B unfavourable is certainly less than this. This work is an encouraging development towards the more precise selection of cases for operative repair with the caveat that nerve repairs do not always work and that it is exceptionally rare to see truly normal function for any nerve repair whether that be done in infancy or in adult life.

Microsurgical techniques in brachial plexus surgery are beyond the scope of this review – the interested reader is referred to the work of Birch and others.[1,18,23] The procedures required in each case are established at direct exploration of the injured plexus and include direct nerve repair, grafting between the two ends of the ruptured nerve using a graft from the sural nerve or others, and in root avulsion nerve transfer of the root to another nerve within or without the plexus such as the accessory or intercostal nerve. It is important to note that significant recovery may take 9–18 months postoperatively and may continue for many years.

The long term outcomes in 24 group IV cases was reported by Anand and Birch.[31] Repair of the plexus was performed in 20 of these 24 infants. Only 3 from 120 spinal nerves were intact, there were 47 avulsions and 58 ruptures. Quantitative measures of cutaneous sensation and of cholinergic sympathetic recovery were made at 46–121 months from operation. Useful motor hand function was restored in 10 of the 20 operated cases, but sensory function greatly exceeded motor or cholinergic sympathetic recovery. These children show perfect localisation of restored sensation in the dermatomes of avulsed spinal nerves which had been re-innervated by intercostal nerves transferred from remote spinal segments. The degree of plasticity within the immature central nervous system shown by this study may be one factor in the remarkable absence of neuropathic pain in CBP which is quite unlike the situation after a traction lesion in adults.

Results of repair of the nerves in CBP are by no means regularly good. The central nervous system in the neonate is very different from that of adults. The cord fills the cervical canal, the spinal roots emerge at or near to a right angle to it. The transitional zone between central and peripheral nervous tissue is immature. Myelination is incomplete, so that conduction velocity in the full-term neonate is about one-half of that in the adult.[32] The baleful effect of proximal axonotomy upon the parent motor neurone was demonstrated by Dyck et al.[33] who showed that a high proportion of them died after amputation of the lower limb for malignant disease. In some respects, the developing nervous system is more vulnerable to peripheral injury than in the adult. Carlstedt and Culheim provided evidence of the extent of neurotrophic support to motor neurones in the immature nervous system.[34] There is a theoretical risk of inducing further central cell death by resection of a neuroma before grafting, for there is always some regeneration across a post ganglionic rupture in CBP.

SECONDARY RECONSTRUCTION

Posterior subluxation – dislocation

In babies, the diagnosis is made by physical examination. The infant is placed supine, the examiner holds both upper limbs with the elbows flexed to 90° and

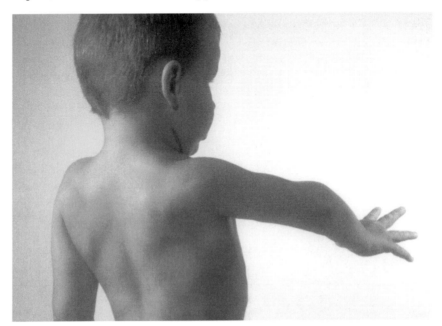

Fig. 6 A 2-year-old boy with partial recovery of a Group II lesion and posterior dislocation of the shoulder – note the prominence of the head of the humerus and the flexion pronation posture of the arm.

the arms are held adducted against the chest before being gentle rotated into lateral rotation. Any loss of passive lateral rotation in the afflicted upper limb is significant. In older children, the posture of the upper limb is characteristic (Fig. 6). The arm lies in medial rotation with flexion and pronation at the elbow. The contour of the shoulder is abnormal, the head is seen and palpated lying behind the glenoid. In nearly every case, a clear impression of the extent of bone deformity can be formed from the physical examination supplemented by plain anterior and posterior axial radiographs. Ultrasound examination is a suitable aid to diagnosis before 12 months of age in those cases where the clinician is suspicious about the congruity of the shoulder.

Treatment for the established disorder is operative and it is probably best done when neurological recovery has matured and when the child is able to walk.[24] This probably interferes rather less with the child's development and reduces the burden upon parents from immobilisation in a plaster of Paris jacket, which includes the arm, but is essential after open reduction. The operation itself is of necessity an extensive one, it includes elongation of contracted muscles and other soft tissue structures, rebalancing of muscle forces across the shoulder and correction by osteotomy of bone deformities.

Musculo-tendinus transfers for wrist and hand function

Muscle transfers are done to rebalance joints and in the growing skeleton to prevent deformity. It is all too easy to replace one deformity such as wrist flexion by another, wrist hyper-extension. To be successful, a muscle transfer must involve plasticity or re-organisation of the somato-sensory cortex and these operations will certainly fail if they are performed too early before neurological recovery is complete. Experienced and skilful occupational

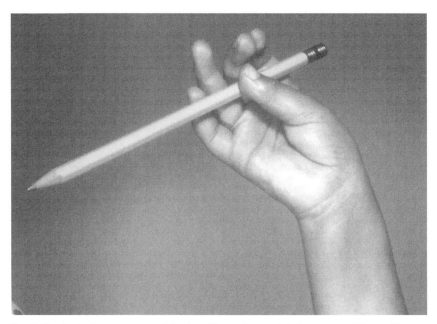

Fig. 7 The typical appearance of the hand in an incompletely recovered Group III lesion – note impaired wrist extension and thumb function, and ulnar deviation of the wrist.

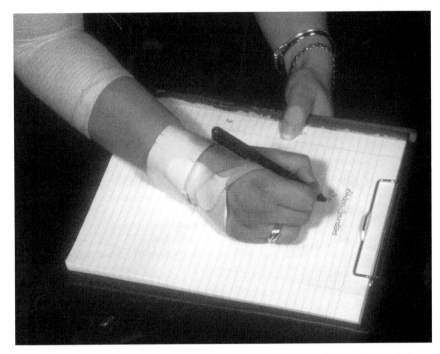

Fig. 8 Simple static splinting of the wrist and thumb enhancing the precision grip in an incompletely recovered Group III lesion.

therapists are essential for success in this field of work. First, they can provide valuable insights into functional defects and also into the adaptations made by the child so that it may in fact be wrong to interfere with the functional pattern that has evolved. Next the provision of simple functional orthoses gives an indication of the benefit of the proposed muscle transfer and is of course the mainstay of postoperative care. Such orthoses may so enhance recovery that planned muscle transfer for restoration of extension of wrist or opposition of thumb proves unnecessary (Figs 7 and 8).

Key points for clinical practice

- The incidence of congenital brachial palsy in the UK and Eire is approximately 1 in 2000 births.

- In a recent population survey in the UK and Eire, risk factors identified were shoulder dystocia, high birth weight and assisted delivery, whilst the risk of congenital brachial palsy is significantly lower in caesarean section.

- The majority of cases are caused by injury at, or just before birth, with evidence in many cases suggestive of injury occurring as a result of trauma caused by maternal propulsive forces. The occurrence of congenital brachial palsy cannot be taken as *prima facie* evidence of excessive applied traction to the brachial plexus by the midwife or obstetrician.

- Although diagnosis is usually straightforward, the clinician needs to particularly consider bony injuries causing pseudoparalysis in the knowledge that they may also co-exist with congenital brachial palsy and radiographs of the affected limb are recommended as well as a chest X-ray in an infant with respiratory symptoms to exclude phrenic nerve palsy.

- The majority of cases affect the upper trunks of the plexus with a minority having a total 'flail arm'.

- In the recent British Paediatric Surveillance Unit survey, only 52% of 276 cases evaluated at a median age of 23 weeks had fully recovered with no cases with a total flail arm making a full recovery.

- Physiotherapy to maintain joint function and muscle strength is the mainstay of treatment in the first weeks of life.

- The place and timing of nerve repair surgery is constrained by difficulties in the selection of those infants who will benefit. There is an emerging consensus that infants with a total flail arm with incomplete recovery at 1 month, and infants with less extensive lesions with incomplete recovery at 3 months, should be referred for specialist assessment.

- Congenital brachial palsy is a potentially disabling condition and the authors strongly recommend the designation of two or three specialist centres in the UK for the assessment and treatment of all but the most mildly affected cases where also research into the role of investigations including neuro-imaging and neurophysiology, the place of nerve repair surgery in the less extensive lesions and other aspects can be meaningfully conducted. Further, these centres would provide the necessary multidisciplinary expertise for the monitoring, prevention and treatment of the potential long-term and disabling secondary complications of congenital brachial palsy that can occur.

References

1. Kay SPJ. Obstetrical brachial palsy. *Br J Plast Surg* 1998; **51**: 43–50.
2. Kay SPJ. Brachial palsies from obstetric procedures. *Lancet* 1999; **354**: 614–615.
3. Narakas AO. Obstetrical brachial plexus injuries. In: Lamb DW. (ed) *The Paralysed Hand*. Edinburgh: Churchill Livingstone, 1987; 116–135.
4. Blaauw G, Slooff A, Muhlig RS. Results of surgery after breech delivery. In: Gilbert A. (ed) *Brachial Plexus Injuries*. London: Dunitz, 2001; 217–225.
5. Slooff ACJ, Blaauw G. Some aspects of obstetrical brachial plexus lesions. In: Alnot JY, Narakas A. (eds) *Traumatic Brachial Plexus Injuries*. Paris: Expansion Scientifique Francaise, 1996; 265–267.
6. Evans-Jones G, Kay SPJ, Weindling AM, Cranny G, Ward A, Bradshaw A, Hernon C. Congenital brachial palsy: incidence, causes, and outcome in the United Kingdom and Republic of Ireland. *Arch Dis Child* 2003; **88**: F185–F189.
7. Adler JB, Patterson RL. Erb's palsy: long term results of treatment in 88 cases. *J Bone Joint Surg (Am)* 1967; **49**: 1052–1064.

8. Roberts L. Shoulder dystocia. In: Studd J. (ed) *Progress in Obstetrics and Gynaecology*, vol. 11. Edinburgh: Churchill Livingstone, 1994; 201–216.

9. Sandmire HF, De Mott RK. Erb's palsy: concepts of causation. *Obstet Gynecol* 2000; **95**: 941–942.

10. Christofferson M, Rydhstreom H. Shoulder dystocia and brachial plexus injury: a population based study. *Gynecol Obstet Invest* 2002; **53**: 42–47.

11. Clements RV. Editorial: Shoulder dystocia. *Clin Risk* 2002; **8**: 215–217.

12. Jennet RJ, Tarby TJ, Kreinick CJ. Brachial plexus palsy: an old problem revisited. *Am J Obstet Gynecol* 1992; **166**: 1673–1677.

13. Gherman RB, Ouzounian JG, Murphy Goodwin T. Brachial plexus palsy: an *in utero* injury? *Am J Obstet Gynecol* 1999; **180**: 1303–1307.

14. Al-Qattan MM, El-Sayed AAF, Al-Kharfy TM, Al-Jurayyan NAM. Obstetrical brachial plexus injury in newborn babies delivered by caesarean section. *J Hand Surg (Br)* 1996; **21**: 263–265.

15. Gonik B, Walker A, Grimm M. Mathematic modelling of forces associated with shoulder dystocia: a comparison of endogenous and exogenous sources. *Am J Obstet Gynecol* 2000; **182**: 689–691.

16. Department of Health. *NHS Maternity Statistics, England: 1989–90 to 1994–1995. Statistical bulletin.* London: Department of Health, 1997.

17. Hageman G, Ramaekers VT, Hilhorst BGJ, Rozeboom AR. Congenital cervical spinal muscular atrophy: a non-familial, non-progressive condition of the upper limbs. *J Neurol Neurosurg Psychiatry* 1993; **56**: 365–368.

18. Birch R. Obstetrical brachial plexus palsy. In: Birch R, Bonney G, Wynne Parry CB. (eds) *Surgical Disorders of the Peripheral Nerves*. Edinburgh: Churchill Livingstone, 1998; 212–225.

19. Bennett GC, Harrold AJ. Prognosis and early management of birth injuries to the brachial plexus. *BMJ* 1976; **1**: 1520–1521.

20. Gilbert A, Razaboni R, Amar-Khodja S. Indications and results of brachial plexus surgery in obstetrical palsy. *Orthop Clin North Am* 1988; **19**: 91–105.

21. Michelow BJ, Clarke HM, Curtis CG et al. The natural history of obstetrical brachial plexus palsy. *Plast Reconstr Surg* 1994; **93**: 675–680.

22. Dodds SD, Wolfe SW. Perinatal brachial plexus palsy. *Curr Opin Paediatr* 2000; **12**: 40–47.

23. Shenaq SM, Berzin G, Lee R, Laurent SP, Nath R, Nelson MR. Brachial plexus birth injuries and current management. *Clin Plast Surg* 1998; **25**: 527–536.

24. Birch R. Medial rotation contracture and posterior dislocation of the shoulder. In: Gilbert A. (ed) *Brachial Plexus Injuries*. London: Dunitz, 2001; 249–259.

25. Gilbert A. Results of repair to the obstetrical brachial plexus. In: Gilbert A. (ed) *Brachial Plexus Injuries*. London: Dunitz, 2001; 211–217.

26. Sjoberg I, Erichs K, Bjerre I. Cause and effect of obstetric (neonatal) brachial plexus palsy. *Acta Paediatr Scand* 1988; **77**: 357–364.

27. Gilbert A. Long term evaluation of brachial plexus surgery in obstetrical palsy. *Hand Clin* 1995; **11**: 583–594.

28. Waters PM. Comparison of the natural history, the outcome of microsurgical repair, and the outcome of operative reconstruction in brachial plexus birth palsy. *J Bone Joint Surg (Am)* 1999; **81**: 649–659.

29. Smith SJM. The role of neurophysiological investigation in traumatic brachial plexus lesions in adults and children. *J Hand Surg (Br)* 1996; **21**: 145–147.

30. Bisinella G, Birch R, Smith SJM. Neurophysiological predictions of outcome in obstetric lesions of the brachial plexus. *J Hand Surg (Br)* 2003; **28**: 148–152.

31. Anand P, Birch R. Restoration of sensory function and lack of long-term chronic pain syndromes after brachial plexus injury in human neonates. *Brain* 2002; **125**: 113–122.

32. Payan J. Clinical electromyography in infancy and childhood. In: Brett EM. (ed) *Paediatric Neurologyr*. Edinburgh: Churchill Livingstone, 1991; 797–829.

33. Dyck PJ, Nukada H, Lais CA, Karnes J. Permanent axonotomy: a model of chronic neuronal degeneration produced by axonal atrophy, myelin remodelling and regeneration. In: Dyck PH, Thomas PK, Lambert EH, Bunge RWB. (eds) *Peripheral Neuropathy*. Philadelphia, PA: Saunders, 1984; 660–690.

34. Carlstedt T, Culheim S. Spinal cord motor neurone maintenance, injury and repair. *Prog Brain Res* 2000; **127**: 501–514.

Kathryn Johnson

6

Withdrawal from drugs of addiction in newborn infants

Drug misuse is common within the UK population. In 2002/2003, there were estimated to be close to 141,000 problem drug misusers in treatment.[1] Statistics suggest approximately 1 in 4 of these are women, of whom 98% are of child bearing age (16–44 years).[2] It can, therefore, be predicted that a significant number of pregnant women are misusing drugs and, as a result, a significant number of infants are exposed to these substances *in utero*. This theory is supported by the currently available data. Anonymous urine screening of greater than 800 pregnant women, attending a UK antenatal clinic, has shown up to 16% had positive screens for one or more illicit substances (Table 1).[3] Meconium screening of newborn infants in a high-risk American population showed even higher levels of exposure with 44% of infants testing positive for opioid, cocaine or cannabis (Table 1).[4] However, caution must be used when interpreting results from the US as the pattern of care for pregnant drug using women and the substances used may vary considerably from the UK.

Urine screening of pregnant women (or their offspring) can have a high rate of false negative results as it is dependent not only on substances reaching a threshold level in the urine but also the time elapsed since the substance was last used. In meconium, metabolites of substances used during pregnancy accumulate as a result of ingestion of amniotic fluid and direct deposition from bile. As meconium is not usually excreted antenatally, and accumulates from the 2nd trimester onwards, its composition does not just reflect recent drug use. Currently, meconium screening is not routinely used in the UK and is considerably more expensive than urine screening. A combination of maternal self report and urine screening may be the most cost effective method of identifying exposed infants as maternal self report alone has been shown to be ineffective.[5]

Kathryn Johnson MBChB
Neonatal Specialist Registrar, Peter Congdon Neonatal Intensive Care Unit, Clarendon Wing, C Floor, Leeds General Infirmary, Leeds LS2 9NS, UK
E-mail: kathrynjohnson@postmaster.co.uk

Table 1 Drug use in pregnancy – maternal and infant screening

	Sherwood et al.[3] Urine screening of pregnant women	Ostrea et al.[4] Meconium screening of newborn infants
Number screened	807	3010
Cannabis (%)	14.5	11.5
Opioids (%)	1.4	20.5
Cocaine (%)	0.4	30.7
1 or more substances (%)	15.6	44.3

Data are expressed as the percentage of the population in which the substances were detected.

PREGNANCY OUTCOME

Illicit drug use during pregnancy can have a wide range of detrimental effects on the developing fetus. Specific effects will depend on the stage of pregnancy, level of exposure and the specific effects of individual substances.

GROWTH AND DEVELOPMENT

Congenital malformations have been associated with the use, during pregnancy of amphetamine[6] and benzodiazepines.[7] The use of opioids during pregnancy has not been shown to increase the risk of malformation.[8] Cocaine use is associated with a variety of congenital abnormalities including cardiac anomalies, limb reduction defects, cloacal abnormalities, intestinal atresia, cerebral infarcts and micropthalmia.[9] These abnormalities may be secondary to the vasoconstrictive effects on both the placental and fetal blood vessels.

Cocaine or multiple drug use has the greatest effect in reducing birth-weight and head circumference.[5] The use of methadone and heroin during pregnancy has been shown in meta-analyses to cause a mean reduction in birth-weight of approximately 500 g.[10]

Cannabis is the most commonly used illicit substance during pregnancy.[3] The potential effects of cannabis on the fetus are controversial, although it has been associated with a significant reduction in gestational age and birth-weight.[3] Much of the controversy results from the difficulty in separating the detrimental effects of tobacco use during pregnancy from the detrimental effects of cannabis use, as half of drug users (compared with 11% of non-users) smoked heavily during pregnancy this can be difficult.[11] Heavy alcohol use, like tobacco use, is seen more commonly in drug users than non-users[11] and is associated with a wide range of detrimental effects on the fetus.

The negative effects on pregnancy of tobacco and alcohol use and the adverse social factors often associated with drug use are very difficult to separate from the direct effects of the particular drugs themselves.

The direct drug effects combined with the associated adverse pregnancy environment work together to increase the likelihood of pregnancy complications.

LABOUR AND DELIVERY

Premature rupture of the membranes, meconium-stained liquor and fetal distress are seen more frequently in the infants of drug users.[4] Opiate has been shown to increase the risk of antepartum haemorrhage and cocaine is particularly associated with placental abruption.[12]

CARE OF THE PREGNANT DRUG USER

Heroin (diamorphine) used to be the most commonly used opioid during pregnancy, now methadone is more commonly used.[13] The majority of women taking methadone are enrolled in methadone programmes, and are reported to have better antenatal care than those not enrolled in such programmes. This improved antenatal care is then associated with a potentially better pregnancy outcome.[14] Methadone has less effect in reducing birth-weight than heroin and also results in a lower neonatal mortality rate.[10] For these reasons, substitution of heroin for methadone during pregnancy is appropriate in order to maintain contact with antenatal services and improve pregnancy outcome.

Cocaine use should be stopped: if not, it should be reduced as much as possible. Benzodiazepines, in view of their significant potential for teratogenecity, should be stopped wherever possible.

The complex care of the pregnant drug user should ideally be provided by designated antenatal clinics, designed specifically for the needs of these women. Unfortunately, at the present time, only about 25% of maternity units provide such a service.[15] These clinics can provide antenatal care together with substance use treatment, in addition to addressing other such issues as nutrition, housing and mental health (up to 10% of pregnant drug users have mental health problems).[16]

NEONATAL OUTCOME

The effects of drug use during pregnancy can be seen both in the short term during the neonatal period and later during childhood.

NEONATAL ABSTINENCE SYNDROME

Drug use (particularly opioid use) during pregnancy can be associated with withdrawal symptoms soon after birth, termed neonatal abstinence syndrome. Neonatal abstinence syndrome may require prolonged pharmacological treatment leading to a long hospital stay[17,18] impacting negatively both on bed occupancy and maternal/infant bonding. Neonatal abstinence syndrome can account for up to 20% of Special Care Baby Unit (SCBU) admissions in some units.[19] The characteristic signs of neonatal abstinence syndrome are listed in Table 2.

Neonatal abstinence syndrome requiring treatment has also been described with the use of benzodiazepines[18] and barbiturates.[20] Cocaine, whilst not physically addictive, causes more severe withdrawal effects in infants exposed to both opioid and cocaine, as compared to those exposed to opioid alone.[11] It has been reported that about 80% of pregnant opioid users are using additional

Table 2 Characteristic signs of neonatal abstinence syndrome

Respiratory system	
	Tachypnoea
Central nervous system	
	Tremors
	Irritability
	Hypertonicity
	Seizures
Gastrointestinal system	
	Poor feeding
	Poor weight gain
	Vomiting
	Diarrhoea
Other	
	Sweating
	Nasal stuffiness
	Fever
	Mottling

substances, of whom one-third are using cocaine;[21] therefore, the potential for significant morbidity from neonatal abstinence syndrome is high.

ASSESSMENT OF NEONATAL ABSTINENCE SYNDROME

Many maternity units have protocols recommending drug-exposed infants are observed for signs of neonatal abstinence syndrome for at least 5 days after delivery. However, research has shown the majority of infants requiring treatment develop signs of neonatal abstinence syndrome with the first 2 days of life.[17]

The effect of maternal methadone dose on the incidence and severity of neonatal abstinence syndrome is controversial; some authors report increasing incidence of neonatal abstinence syndrome with increasing methadone dose, others report no such link.[14,19,21] Reduction of maternal methadone dosage during pregnancy should be cautious as over-enthusiastic dose reductions may lead to withdrawal symptoms in the mother and the risk of illicit additional drug use.

Assessment of the severity of neonatal abstinence syndrome, and the potential need for treatment is achieved in most units by the use of scoring charts. A wide variety of scoring charts are used in the UK from simple charts in which three signs are deemed to be present or absent, to the Finnegan chart, a complex 22-point scoring chart requiring a subjective assessment of a wide variety of signs in the infant.[22] The Finnegan chart is now the most commonly used in the UK[15] and is one of the few charts to have been validated, having been shown to reduce treatment duration when compared with subjective assessment alone.[22] Very few other scoring charts have been validated.

Guidance must be given as to when throughout the day scoring should be performed as many normal infants may score highly, for example, before a feed.

Overall, the positive impact of the use of scoring charts in the treatment of neonatal abstinence syndrome is supported by very limited evidence. Such charts can require a considerable amount of nursing time and expertise to complete correctly although their use does allow practice to be standardised within hospitals and allows clear treatment protocols based on specific scores to be drawn up.

Recent work using movement (recorded on a portable motion detector) as a measure of severity of withdrawal has produced encouraging results.[23] This method may allow for a more simple and objective (computer generated) measure of withdrawal and has been validated both against traditional scoring systems and when compared with non-withdrawing controls.

TREATMENT OF NEONATAL ABSTINENCE SYNDROME

Prior to commencing treatment for neonatal abstinence syndrome, alternative diagnoses for withdrawal symptoms must be excluded by thorough clinical examination and appropriate laboratory investigation.

Up to 80% of infants exposed to opioid *in utero* have neonatal abstinence syndrome severe enough to require pharmacological treatment.[24] The decision to commence pharmacological treatment is usually based on repeated high scores on the scoring chart. Once the decision to start treatment has been made, there is limited available evidence to inform practice as to which is the most appropriate agent to use. Pharmacological agents used in the UK and their frequency of use are listed in Table 3.

The rationale for the use of opioids to treat neonatal abstinence syndrome is based on their specific neurochemical effects, treating the abnormalities in the brain induced by opioid withdrawal. Sedative agents (chlorpromazine, choral hydrate, diazepam, phenobarbitone) act non-specifically to sedate and reduce the manifestations of neonatal abstinence syndrome. Although chloral hydrate is used in some units, there is no evidence to support such practice. Chlorpromazine was previously the most commonly prescribed agent in neonatal abstinence syndrome;[25] however, there is only one small trial to support its use.[26] UK practice has now changed to favour the use of an opioid as the treatment of choice;[15] this is supported by the available evidence. Much of the available evidence is from older, poorly designed, non-randomised trials; more recent evidence, however, continues to support the use of an opioid as the treatment of choice.[19]

Many of the older trials comparing pharmacological treatments for neonatal abstinence syndrome have used the opioid preparation paregoric. This substance is no longer in use as additives in the preparation included camphor, alcohol and

Table 3 Pharmacological treatment options for neonatal abstinence syndrome and their frequency of use in the UK [*n* = number of SCBU units responding to the survey].

Pharmacological agent	UK units using agent as first-line treatment (%)	
	1994 (*n* = 179)	2002 (*n* = 182)
Opioid (morphine, methadone, diamorphine)	10.8	80
Chlorpromazine	70.8	6
Chloral hydrate	7.7	9
Diazepam	1.5	0
Phenobarbitone	9.2	4

benzoic acid. In the majority of UK units, the opioid used is morphine; methadone is very occasionally used and may confer certain advantages over morphine including a longer duration of action allowing the potential for a once daily dose. This single daily dose may make discharge on treatment more practical. There are no trials directly comparing the efficacy of morphine versus methadone in the treatment of neonatal abstinence syndrome.

The available evidence does mainly concentrate on the treatment of neonatal abstinence syndrome secondary to opioid withdrawal. Many infants have significant polydrug exposure and there is little information on the treatment of such infants. Opioid treatment alone may not be as effective in these infants; in up to 50% of cases a second line agent may be required. Higher maternal methadone doses may also increase the likelihood of the need for a second-line agent.[19]

There is no evidence to inform practice as to which is the most appropriate starting dose of morphine when commencing treatment for neonatal abstinence syndrome. A total daily dose of up to 0.5 mg/kg is frequently used, divided into 3–6 doses depending on individual neonatal unit protocol. Comparisons of the different dosing and frequency regimens for morphine are needed to determine the most appropriate treatment schedule. Once symptoms or score are under control, the dose of morphine can be reduced, usually initially by reducing the dose, and then by reducing the frequency of doses. In the more severely affected infants, dose reductions as small as 10% at a time may be required. The dose of morphine should not be reduced unless the infant's symptoms or score have been stable for at least 48 h in order to avoid a rebound increase in symptoms. There is no evidence to suggest what the safe maximum dose of morphine is in infants with neonatal abstinence syndrome; doses above 0.5 mg/kg/day may sometimes be required.

DISCHARGE AND FOLLOW UP FROM THE SPECIAL CARE BABY UNIT

Once treatment is commenced, it can be weaned according to scores until it can be discontinued. Treatment is frequently prolonged; recent work has shown the median duration of treatment in neonatal abstinence syndrome to be 29 days.[17] Hospital stay may then need to be extended, once treatment has stopped, for non-medical reasons.[27] About a quarter of units in the UK discharge infants on treatment if social circumstances are appropriate, thus reducing bed occupancy and improving maternal/infant bonding.[15] Although discharge on treatment will address the problems both of bed occupancy and bonding, it is not without difficulty as failure to attend out patient follow-up appointments in this population can be as high as 50%.[27] With appropriate specialised multidisciplinary follow-up of infants discharged on treatment, the clinic attendance rate can be over 90%;[28] however, this type of specialised multidisciplinary follow-up can be extremely labour intensive. Follow-up is not only important in view of neonatal abstinence syndrome and its treatment, but also in view of the multiple potential adverse pregnancy outcomes associated with maternal drug use during pregnancy.

In addition, serological follow-up may be important in those infants born to HIV or hepatitis C positive mothers. Those born to hepatitis B positive mothers should have vaccination prior to discharge.

BREAST FEEDING

Breast feeding should be encouraged in methadone using women, apart from those who are HIV positive. The amount of methadone excreted in breast milk is small, even at high maternal doses.[29] As a result, there should be no dose limitation as to which mothers can breast feed. Those choosing to breast feed should be advised not to stop suddenly, as the sudden cessation of a small amount of opiate in the breast milk can lead to the appearance of withdrawal symptoms.[30] In women who are using other substances, the advice regarding breast feeding is variable. Hepatitis C is not a contra-indication to breast feeding.[31]

CHILDHOOD OUTCOME

GROWTH

Some catch-up growth of infants exposed to methadone *in utero* has been shown during the first 12 months of life although infants did remain small.[32] Poor growth in the first months of life may in part reflect the poor feeding associated with neonatal abstinence syndrome;[33] however, this association is contradicted in other studies which report an association between hyperphagia and excessive weight gain in infants with neonatal abstinence syndrome.[34] Growth may also be affected by medical problems such as respiratory tract infections reportedly more frequent in children of drug users[35] and the on-going medical problems associated with any of the adverse birth/neonatal events seen more frequently in these infants.

Infants of drug using mothers are more likely to have head circumference measurements below the 3rd centile, persistent at least until 18 months of age.[35]

DEVELOPMENT

Some children will have on-going developmental problems, linked specifically to the direct effects of a particular drug, for example, maternal cocaine use leading to cerebral infarction and subsequent cerebral palsy.

Studies of developmental outcome in drug-exposed infants and children vary widely in their results. This reflects the on-going difficulties in studying this population including difficulties in finding appropriately matched controls, poor compliance with long-term follow-up, a wide variety of drugs of exposure and a wide variety of developmental tests available. Differences may also result from comparisons in some studies with matched or semi-matched controls and in others comparisons with general population norms.

It has been reported that up to 85% of drug-exposed infants require follow-up of neurodevelopmental or behavioural problems.[16] Other studies report no defects in some aspects of development but on-going defects in other skill areas including, cognition, behaviour and language, throughout the first 5 years of life.[25] Assessing the effects on cognition specifically, when reviewing studies using a standardised test (the Bayley scales of infant development) differences with the non-drug exposed population appear over time. At 6 and 12 months, no differences in development when drug-exposed infants were compared with matched controls were seen.[36,37] At 18 months, Bayley scales have been reported to be significantly lower than matched controls.[35] By the time the children reach 3 years of age, only 20% in one large study were reported to have scores within the normal range. At 3–6 years, slightly more of the same children had a developmental assessment within the normal range.[16] However, the comparisons were made against population norms rather than matched controls.

On-going problems with behaviour and language may reflect the poor stimulation the infants and children may receive in the home environment.

SOCIAL CIRCUMSTANCES

It has been suggested that complex social circumstances add in excess of 1 week on an infant's stay on the SCBU once medical treatment has ceased.[27] It must be decided whilst an infant is on the SCBU whether or not they will be discharged with their mother. Up to 50% of drug-exposed infants have older siblings not in the care of the mother.[17] Ideally, prebirth planning meetings should be held to address any social issues that may arise after the delivery of the infant. During such meetings, a provisional plan both for the immediate post-natal period and for discharge can be formulated. Such planning meetings may be best facilitated when specific antenatal clinics for drug-using women exist.

In the US, there has been a trend away from drug-exposed infants being discharged with their mothers towards fostering and adoption.[16] Some authors suggest that fostering does not necessarily protect from the adverse developmental and behavioural outcomes potentially seen in these infants.[38] Significant central nervous system abnormalities have been shown in older children, both in those exposed to drugs *in utero* and those not exposed *in utero* but living with drug-using parents suggesting at least to some degree some developmental defects could be related to the adverse social environment.[39] In some cases, fostering may protect from disruption in home life such as emergency child care measures required when a parent is remanded in custody; almost two-thirds of infants born to drug using mothers have previously been incarcerated.[40]

Children at home with drug-using parents may be at increased risk of abuse and neglect. In one series, two-thirds of children taken into care in the US as a result of maltreatment were children of substance users.[41] These findings are supported by other work, again in the US, suggesting one-third of children exposed to drugs *in utero* were being neglected or abused.[42]

Whether or not the child remains in the care of his/her mother, extra support and regular contact with a wide variety of health care professionals is essential. As only 50% of these infants return for follow-up, this can be problematic. Intensive support of drug-using mothers at home can improve both out patient attendance and outcome.[40]

Given the risks of developmental, behavioural and emotional problems in children of drug users and the associated risks of abuse and neglect, encouraging parents to undergo detoxification may be appropriate. Residential programmes for both drug users and their offspring can result in abstinence from drugs in some parents,[43] and minimise disruption to families as compared with detoxification programmes admitting the parents only. However, such programmes can be expensive and whether this detoxification has any positive effect on behaviour and development has not be studied.

Key points for clinical practice

- Drug use amongst pregnant women is common.

- Patterns of drug use may vary across the UK and from country to country.

- Research in this area is fraught with methodological difficulties and evidence must be interpreted with this is mind. Much of the research has been carried in the US where the patterns and treatment of drug use differ; therefore, results must be applied to the UK population with a degree of caution.

- Cocaine, amphetamine and benzodiazepines can cause fetal malformation.

- Drug use during pregnancy is associated with a wide range of pregnancy and labour complications.

- Newborn infants can display withdrawal symptoms as a result of the development of physical dependency *in utero* – neonatal abstinence syndrome.

- Neonatal abstinence syndrome is most commonly seen following maternal opioid use during pregnancy.

- Up to 80% of infants exposed to opioid *in utero* (either alone or with other substances) will require pharmacological treatment for neonatal abstinence syndrome; treatment may be prolonged.

- The limited available evidence suggests an opioid is the most effective treatment for neonatal abstinence syndrome.

- Methadone rather than heroin use during pregnancy leads to improved antenatal attendance and pregnancy outcome; however, its use associated with more severe neonatal abstinence syndrome.

- The potential long-term detrimental effects of drug use during pregnancy on development and behaviour are varied, ascribing these effects directly to drugs used during pregnancy is difficult.

- Fostering and adoption has not been consistently shown to confer any advantage on development and behaviour.

References

1. Department of Health. *Provisional Statistics. National Drug Treatment Monitoring system in England. 2002/2003*. London: Department of Health, 2003.
2. Department of Health. *Regional Drug Misuse Database. 6 months ending March 2001*. London: Department of Health, 2001.

3. Sherwood RA, Keating J, Kavvadia V, Greenough A, Peters TJ. Substance misuse in early pregnancy and relationship to fetal outcome. *Eur J Pediatr* 1999; **158**: 488–492.
4. Ostrea EM, Brady M, Gause S, Raymundo AL, Stevens M. Drug screening of newborns by meconium analysis: a large scale prospective, epidemiologic study. *Pediatrics* 1992; **89**: 107–113.
5. Gillogley KM, Evans AT, Hansen RL, Samuels SJ, Batra KK. The perinatal impact of cocaine, amphetamine and opiate use detected by universal intrapartum screening. *Am J Obstet Gynecol* 1990; **163**: 1535–1542.
6. Eriksson M, Zetterstrom R. The effect of amphetamine-addiction on the fetus and child. *Teratology* 1981; **24/2**: 39A.
7. Laegreid L, Olegard R, Walstrom JNC, Conradi N. Teratogenic effects of benzodiazepine use during pregnancy. *J Pediatr* 1989; **114**: 126–131.
8. Ostrea EM, Chavez CJ. Perinatal problems (excluding neonatal withdrawal) in maternal drug addiction: a study of 830 cases. *J Pediatr* 1979; **94**: 292–295.
9. Rizk B, Atterbury JL, Groome L. Reproductive risks of cocaine. *Hum Reprod Update* 1996; **2**: 43–55.
10. Hulse GK, Milne E, English DR, Holman CDJ. The relationship between maternal use of heroin and methadone and infant birthweight. *Addiction* 1997; **92**: 1571–1579.
11. Bada HS, Bauer CR, Shankaran S *et al.* Central and autonomic system signs with *in utero* drug exposure. *Arch Dis Child* 2002; **87**: F106–F112.
12. Hulse GK, Milne E, English DR, Holman CDJ. Assessing the relationship between maternal opiate use and antepartum haemorrhage. *Addiction* 1998; **93**: 1553–1558.
13. Lissauer T, Ghaus K, Rivers RPA. Maternal drug abuse: effects on the child. *Curr Paediatr* 1994; **4**: 235–239.
14. Suffet F, Brotman R. A comprehensive care programme for pregnant addicts: obstetrical, neonatal, and child development outcomes. *Int J Addict* 1984; **19**: 199–219.
15. Johnson K, Greenough A, Gerada C. Survey of antenatal and neonatal management of drug abuse. *Br J Intensive Care* 2003; **Summer**: 43–45.
16. Budden SS. Intrauterine exposure to drugs and alcohol: how do the children fare? *Medscape General Medicine* [eJournal www.medscape.com], 1999; 1(1).
17. Johnson K, Greenough A, Gerada C. Maternal drug use and length of neonatal unit stay. *Addiction* 2003; **98**: 785–789.
18. Coghlan D, Milner M, Clarke T *et al.* Neonatal abstinence syndrome. *Ir Med J* 1999; **92**: 232–233.
19. Jackson L, Ting A, McKay S, Galea P, Skeoch C. A randomised controlled trial of morphine versus phenobarbitone for neonatal abstinence syndrome. *Arch Dis Child* 2004; **89**: F300–F304.
20. Blumenthal I, Lindsay S. Neonatal barbiturate withdrawal. *Postgrad Med J* 1977; **53**: 157–158.
21. Brown HL, Britton KA, Mahaffey D *et al.* Methadone maintenance in pregnancy: a reappraisal. *Am J Obstet Gynecol* 1998; **179**: 459–463.
22. Finnegan LP, Connaughton JF, Kron RE, Emich JP. Neonatal abstinence syndrome: assessment and management. *Additive Dis* 1975; **2**: 141–158.
23. O'Brien C, Hunt R, Jeffrey HE. Measurement of movement is an objective method to assist in assessment of opiate withdrawal in newborns. *Arch Dis Child* 2004; **89**: F305–F309.
24. van Baar AL, Soepatmi S, Gunning WB, Akkerhuis GW. Development after prenatal exposure to cocaine, heroin and methadone. *Acta Paediatr Suppl* 1994; **404**: 40–46.
25. Morrison CL, Siney C. A survey of the management of neonatal opiate withdrawal in England and Wales. *Eur J Pediatr* 1996; **155**: 323–326.
26. Kahn E, Neumann L, Polk GA. The course of heroin withdrawal syndrome in newborn infants treated with phenobarbitol or chlorpromazine. *Pediatrics* 1969; **75**: 495–500.
27. Payot A, Berner M. Hospital stay and short-term follow up of children of drug-abusing mothers born in an urban community hospital – a retrospective review. *Eur J Pediatr* 2000; **159**: 679–683.
28. Oei J, Feller J-M. Coordinated outpatient care of the narcotic dependent infant. *J Paediatr Child Health* 2001; **37**: 266–270.
29. Wojnar-Horton RE, Kristensen JH, Yapp P *et al.* Methadone distribution and excretion

into breast milk of clients in a methadone maintenance programme. *Br J Clin Pharmacol* 1997; **44**: 543–547.

30. Malpas TJ, Darlow BA. Neonatal abstinence syndrome following abrupt cessation of breast feeding. *NZ Med J* 1999; **112**: 12–13.

31. European Paediatric Hepatitis C Virus Network. Effects of mode of delivery and infant feeding on the risk of mother-to-child transmission of hepatitis C virus. *Br J Obstet Gynaecol* 2001; **108**: 371–377.

32. Vance JC, Chant DC, Tudehope DI, Gray PH, Hayes AJ. Infants born to narcotic dependent mothers: physical growth patterns in the first 12 months of life. *J Pediatr Child Health* 1997; **33**: 504–508.

33. Weinberger SM, Kandall SR, Doberczak TM, Thornton JC, Bernstein J. Early weight change patterns in neonatal abstinence. *Am J Dis Child* 1986; **140**: 829–832.

34. Shephard R, Greenough A, Johnson K, Gerada C. Hyperphagia, weight gain and neonatal drug withdrawal. *Eur J Pediatr* 2002; **91**: 951–953.

35. Rosen TS, Johnson HL. Children of methadone maintained mothers: follow up to 18 months of age. *J Pediatr* 1982; **101**: 192–196.

36. Van Baar AL, Fleury P, Ultee CA. Behaviour in first year of life after drug dependent pregnancy. *Arch Dis Child* 1989; **64**: 241–245.

37. Kaltenbach K, Finnegan LP. Perinatal and developmental outcome of infants exposed to methadone *in utero. Neurtoxicol Teratol* 1987; **9**: 311–313.

38. Soepatmi S. Developmental outcomes of children of mothers dependent on heroin or heroin/methadone during pregnancy. *Acta Paediatr Suppl* 1994; **404**: 36–39.

39. Guo X, Spencer JW, Suess PE *et al.* Cognitive brain potential alterations in boys exposed to opiates: *in utero* and lifestyle comparisons. *Addict Behav* 1994; **19**: 429–441.

40. Black MM, Nair P, Kight C *et al.* Parenting and early development among children of drug-abusing women: effects of home intervention. *Pediatrics* 1994; **94**: 440–448.

41. Famularo R, Kinscherff R, Fenton T. Parental substance abuse and the nature of child maltreatment. *Child Abuse Negl* 1992; **16**: 475–483.

42. Jaudes PK, Ekwo E, Van Voorhis J. Association of drug abuse and child abuse. *Child Abuse Negl* 1995; **19**: 1065–1075.

43. Keen J, Oliver P, Rowse G, Mathers N. Keeping families of heroin addicts together: results of 13 months intake for community detoxification and rehabilitation at a family centre for drug users. *Fam Pract* 2000; **17**: 484–489.

Leigh E. Dyet Frances M. Cowan

7

Magnetic resonance imaging of injury to the preterm brain

Infants born prematurely are at increased risk of neurological, cognitive and behavioural difficulties.[1] These include cerebral palsy or minor motor difficulties, impaired intelligence quotient (IQ) and attention deficit hyperactivity disorder. The ability to identify infants at particular risk is an important part of their on-going management so that appropriate information can be provided to parents and also the appropriate support and follow-up can be initiated. Cranial ultrasound has been the mainstay of neonatal cerebral imaging for many years and identifies significant haemorrhagic[2] and cystic lesions[3] with good sensitivity. However, with the increasing use of antenatal steroids and improvements in neonatal intensive care, these abnormalities occur less frequently. The majority of neurodevelopmental problems found in preterm infants no longer relate to these well-defined abnormalities and are more likely to result from subtle cerebral injury or abnormalities in cerebral development.[4] Although cranial ultrasound can identify the majority of echogenic and echolucent lesions that lead to motor deficits and cerebral palsy,[5,6] it does not reliably identify subtle damage seen on magnetic resonance imaging (MRI).[7]

MRI allows comprehensive imaging of the neonatal brain. Areas not well visualised on cranial ultrasound such as the cerebral cortex, extracerebral space and posterior fossa can be imaged and injury to white and grey matter can be seen in detail. MRI allows the brain to be viewed in three-dimensions and cerebral volumes to be quantified. Newer techniques such as diffusion-weighted imaging, tractography and deformation-based morphometry give

Leigh E. Dyet MBBS BMedSci MRCPCH
Clinical Research Fellow, Department of Paediatrics, Obstetrics & Gynaecology, Imperial College London, Weston Laboratory, 1st Floor, IRDB, Hammersmith Hospital, Du Cane Road, London W12 0NN, UK.

Frances M. Cowan MBBS DCH MRCP MRCGP MRCPCH PhD (for correspondence)
Senior Lecturer and Honorary Consultant in Neonatal Neurology, Department of Paediatrics, 5th Floor, Hammersmith House, Hammersmith Hospital, Du Cane Road, London W12 0NN, UK
E-mail: f.cowan@imperial.ac.uk

greater insights into the patterns of injury and the development of the preterm brain in the *ex utero* environment. Despite these advantages, MRI is not available in all neonatal centres, it is expensive and infants require transportation. However, with increasing experience in this field, greater numbers of preterm infants will have a brain MRI as part of their neonatal management. What remains uncertain is the relationship between many of the abnormalities found on MRI and the long-term neurodevelopmental outcome of these infants and this is an area of continuing research.

SAFETY AND EQUIPMENT

Advances in MRI-compatible ventilation, monitoring and transportation equipment allows infants as immature as 23 weeks' gestational age to be imaged safely.[8] MRI-compatible incubators have been developed, often with in-built neonatal head coils to increase signal-to-noise ratio and improve image quality. To avoid image motion artefact, the infant's head must remain still and many institutions achieve this by feeding and wrapping infants and scanning them during natural sleep. The success of this method depends upon the clinical state of the infant and oral sedation can also be used. We use oral chloral hydrate as a sedative, in doses of 30–50 mg/kg. This has proved a safe and effective regimen in association with ear protection (dental putty and Natus MiniMuffs, Natus Medical Inc., San Carlos, CA, USA), swaddling and a bean-bag pillow moulded around the head. We do not use anaesthesia for scanning young infants. Prior to sedation, a thorough respiratory and neurological assessment of the child is made. Infants are kept nil-by-mouth for about 2 h prior to sedative administration depending on their gestation and feeding patterns. The sedative is given just before the scan is due to take place as it works quickly when the infant has an empty stomach. If infection is suspected, an intravenous cannula is inserted prior to imaging so that contrast agent can be injected during the scan. The infant's heart rate and oxygen saturations are monitored throughout scanning and experienced paediatric staff skilled in the transportation and resuscitation of the neonate and also familiar with MRI procedures supervise the imaging. After the scan, more mature infants who have come from home return to the ward for monitoring until they are awake and have taken a feed. If possible, parents are shown the scans on the same day to avoid delays in imparting information. This policy may be less appropriate in different clinical settings. Reports containing the scan findings, likely aetiology, known clinical implications, suggested investigations and the need for repeat scanning are sent out after a scan review meeting.

SCAN ACQUISITION AND SEQUENCES

Imaging of the preterm brain has mainly been carried out on 1 Tesla (T) or 1.5 T MRI scanners; however, 3 T scanners are now available for research. At this higher magnetic field strength, greater detail can be seen partly due to the increased signal-to-noise ratio. T1-weighted and T2-weighted sequences are mainly used to acquire images in these infants. In particular, T2-weighted, fast spin echo sequences provide very good contrast between tissues. The tissue signal intensities using these sequences are shown in Table 1.

Table 1 Signal intensities of tissues using T1- and T2-weighted sequences

	T1-weighted sequences	T2-weighted sequences
Cerebrospinal fluid (CSF)	Low signal intensity (black)	High signal intensity (white)
Myelinated white matter	High signal intensity	Low signal intensity
Unmyelinated white matter	Intermediate signal intensity (dependent on gestational age)	Intermediate signal intensity (dependent on gestational age)
Grey matter	High signal intensity (reduces after term)	Low signal intensity (reduces after term)

Each department undertaking neonatal imaging must have a good understanding of the signal intensities produced by different sequences when imaging the normal neonatal brain. Sequences have to be adapted from those used in adults because of the high water content within the brain in infants. Newer imaging equipment improves image acquisition speed and sequences required for most clinical examinations can be acquired within about 20 minutes. Images can be acquired in the axial, coronal and sagittal planes; however, with newer software, 3-D volume sets can be reformatted into any plane and viewed. The axial view allows good visualisation of the posterior limb of the internal capsule and the basal ganglia and thalamus. The sagittal plane visualises anatomy and gives good views of the corpus callosum, cerebellar vermis and pituitary. The coronal view provides good images of the cerebellum and hippocampus. Images should be acquired in at least two planes using two different sequences. Additional views and sequences depend upon the expected pathology.

NORMAL IMAGING OF THE PRETERM BRAIN

CORTICAL FOLDING

At 24 weeks' gestational age, the brain has a smooth outline and little sulcation and gyration (Fig. 1A). Cortical folding becomes more complex with increasing gestational age as demonstrated by neuropathological and fetal MRI studies. This process continues in the *ex utero* environment if an infant is born prematurely; however, at term equivalent age infants born at < 30 weeks' gestational age have less complex cortical folding and a smaller cortical surface area than their term born peers (Fig. 1B,C).[9] This suggests that prematurity may be detrimental to the normal development of the cerebral cortex.

CEREBRAL VOLUME

Total cerebral volumes have been calculated from serial imaging of infants between 25 and 42 weeks' gestational age.[9] These volumes increase exponentially with increasing gestational age at a rate of 8% per week (95% confidence intervals 7–9%). The mean cerebral volume of preterm infants imaged at term equivalent age does not differ significantly from the cerebral volumes of infants born at term;

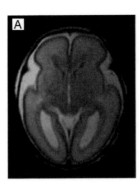 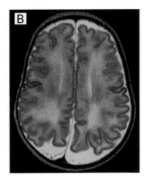 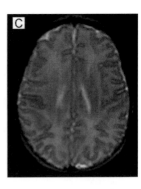

Fig. 1 (A) T2-weighted axial image showing the cortical folding of an infant born at 24 weeks' gestational age and imaged 1 day after birth. (B) T2-weighted axial image showing cortical folding of an infant born at 26 weeks' gestational age and imaged at term equivalent age. (C) T2-weighted axial image showing cortical folding of an infant born at term.

however, their cortical surface area is reduced.[9] Further information about volume changes of specific tissue types is provided using quantitative MRI and tissue segmentation.[10] Unmyelinated white matter is the most abundant tissue type prior to 36 weeks' gestational age with a marked increase in myelinated white matter occurring after this age. The tissue type with the greatest relative increase in volume between 29 and 41 weeks' gestational age is cortical grey matter, possibly due to neuronal differentiation.

WHITE MATTER MATURATION

Serial MRI has allowed the normal process of white matter maturation to be visualised. Until about 29 weeks' gestational age, the white matter in the periventricular regions and the centrum semiovale can be divided into three separate bands with alternating signal intensity characteristics (Fig. 2A).[11] These white matter details are most easily identified on T2-weighted sequences. The inner layer is of high signal intensity and widens with increasing gestational age. The middle layer is of relatively lower signal intensity and is thought to represent an increased density of cells migrating outwards towards the cortex. The sub-cortical layer is high-signal intensity and becomes narrower with increasing gestational age and is difficult to visualise by 29 weeks. This layer may correspond to the cortical subplate. These findings are common to all infants unless there has been significant disruption of white matter development, for example due to haemorrhagic parenchymal infarction or severe post-haemorrhagic hydrocephalus.[11]

White matter bands appear incomplete inferiorly; however, they can still be identified in the anterior and posterior periventricular regions (Fig. 2B). Anteriorly, these areas are described as 'caps' and are more clearly demarcated than the superior bands. Histologically, they correspond to converging fibres from within the white matter. These fibres appear more abundant and less organised than in other regions of white matter.[12] 'Caps' are present on imaging from about 24 weeks' gestational age and are only absent if there is significant white matter disruption. The posterior periventricular areas are

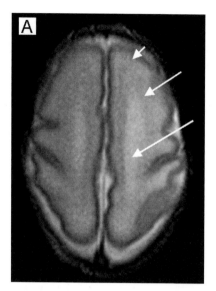 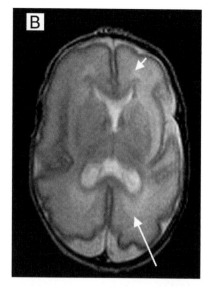

Fig. 2 (A) T2-weighted axial image showing white matter bands in an infant born at 25^{+5} weeks' gestational age and imaged at 29^{+5} weeks' gestational age. Inner layer (long arrow), middle layer (medium arrow) and subcortical layer (short arrow). (B) T2-weighted axial image showing 'caps' (short arrow) and 'arrowheads' (long arrow) in the same infant as in (A).

described as 'arrowheads'. These can also be seen from 24 weeks' gestational age; however, they are sometimes missing from very early images in the most immature infants. 'Arrowheads' are of high-signal intensity on T2-weighted sequences, however 'caps' have additional areas of low-signal intensity. White matter bands, 'caps' and 'arrowheads' are developmental findings and become less obvious from 36 weeks' gestational age.[11] Provisional results from imaing at 3 Tesla suggest that these white matter detals are still visible at later gestations, but these findings need further clarification.

MYELINATION

The identification of myelin within the preterm brain depends upon the type of MRI sequence used, the anatomical site and the gestational age of the infant. In preterm infants, myelin within the grey matter is seen more easily on T2-weighted, fast spin echo imaging, whereas within the white matter tracts it can be seen more clearly on T1-weighted sequences.[13] After term, but within the first year after birth, myelin is more clearly identified on inversion recovery, fast spin echo sequences. In older children, it is better defined using T2-weighted sequences. Myelin can be identified histologically at approximately 25 weeks' gestational age within the posterior brainstem. Using MRI, myelin has been identified in the cerebellar peduncles at about 25 weeks' gestational age. Prior to 28 weeks' gestational age, myelin has been identified within a number of structures including the gracile and cuneate nuclei, cerebellar vermis, dentate nucleus and the medial longitudinal fasciculus. There are no new sites of myelination identified on brain MRI between 28 and 36 weeks' gestational age. After 36 weeks' gestational age, myelin can be identified

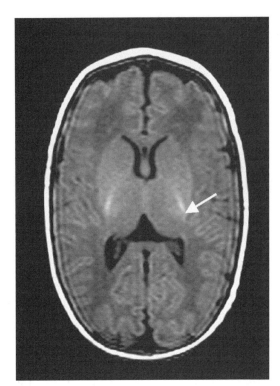

Fig. 3 T1-weighted axial image showing myelination within the posterior part of the posterior limb of the internal capsule (arrow) in an infant born at 30 weeks' gestational age and imaged at term equivalent age.

within the posterior limb of the internal capsule (Fig. 3), the corona radiata, the precentral and postcentral gyri and the lateral geniculate bodies.[13] The progression of myelination within the brain of the preterm infant does not appear to differ significantly from that of the fetus *in utero*.[14] However, some preterm infants develop myelin within the posterior limb of the internal capsule at an earlier gestational age and others have delayed myelination. The significance of premature myelination remains unclear; however, there is evidence that delay in myelination correlates with an adverse neurodevelopmental outcome.[15]

LATERAL VENTRICLES AND EXTRACEREBRAL SPACE

The normal dimensions of the extracerebral space have been studied on MRI scans taken soon after birth in infants born between 29 and 42 weeks' gestational age.[16] There is little variation in its width between infants born at different gestational ages and measurements range between 0–4 mm. The most immature infants can have an increased extracerebral space width in the posterior parietal region that is easily identified in the para-sagittal plane and can measure up to 13 mm. This measurement decreases over time on serial imaging and is not usually seen at term age equivalent. It is, therefore, important not to diagnose cerebral atrophy in infants who are still preterm using this measurement.

Quantitative MRI has been used to calculate cerebrospinal fluid (CSF) volumes within the brain of infants born between 29 and 41 weeks' gestational age.[10] The absolute volume of CSF increases over this age range; however, the

CSF volume relative to total cerebral volume decreases. This suggests that the extracerebral space and ventricular system is smaller in infants born at later gestational ages. This study used single images taken within 2 weeks of birth; however, serial changes in CSF volume have not been published within the preterm population.

BASAL GANGLIA AND THALAMUS

In preterm infants, the signal intensities within the basal ganglia and thalami change with increasing gestational age.[17] On T1-weighted sequences, the basal ganglia are initially seen as high-signal intensity in the most immature infants but, with increasing gestational age, the signal intensity decreases leaving focal high signal within the ventrolateral nucleus of the thalamus, the globus pallidus and the posterior part of the putamen by 35 weeks. Early myelination in the posterior limb of the internal capsule can also be seen as high-signal intensity. On T2-weighted imaging, the thalamus initially has a low signal intensity with the ventrolateral nucleus of the thalamus being particularly prominent. The lentiform nucleus is more heterogeneous. With increasing post-menstrual age, the basal ganglia and thalamus become more iso-intense, but the ventrolateral nucleus of the thalamus and the lateral border of the lentiform nucleus remain of low signal intensity. Early myelination within the posterior part of the posterior limb of the internal capsule can be identified as low-signal intensity on T2-weighted images and at this stage always appears less advanced than on T1-weighted images.

GERMINAL MATRIX

The germinal matrix can be identified as high-signal intensity on T1-weighted sequences and low-signal intensity on T2-weighted sequences. These signal characteristics relate to its high cellularity. It is present from the end of the first trimester in the anterior and lateral margins of the lateral ventricles. At about 29 weeks' gestational age, it begins to involute. At term, only small residual areas remain at the anterolateral angles of the lateral ventricles, adjacent to the head of the caudate nucleus and adjacent to the thalamus.[18]

IMAGING OF PRETERM BRAIN INJURY

GERMINAL LAYER HAEMORRHAGE

Germinal layer haemorrhage within the matrix is of high-signal intensity on T1-weighted sequences and low-signal intensity on T2-weighted sequences depending on the timing of the scan (Fig. 4A).[19] Haemorrhage may still be seen on T2-weighted images several months after the original injury because of the presence of haemosiderin. A germinal layer haemorrhage can be distinguished from the underlying germinal matrix by its irregular borders and asymmetry,[18] and it may also become hypo-intense in comparison on T2-weighted imaging. It is most commonly seen overlying the caudate head, but it can also occur more temporally probably from the remnant of matrix behind the thalamus.

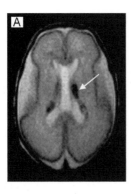
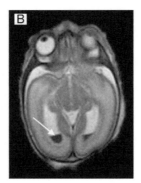
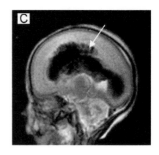

Fig. 4 (A) T2-weighted axial image showing bilateral germinal layer haemorrhages (arrow) in an infant born at 24[+6] weeks' gestational age and imaged at 28[+2] weeks' gestational age. (B) T2-weighted axial image showing bilateral intraventricular haemorrhage with fluid levels in the posterior horns (arrow) in an infant born at 25 weeks' gestational age and imaged 3 days after birth. (C) T2-weighted sagittal image showing a haemorrhagic parenchymal infarction (arrow) in an infant born at 23 weeks' gestational age and imaged 4 days after birth.

INTRAVENTRICULAR HAEMORRHAGE

Intraventricular haemorrhage has the same signal intensity characteristics as germinal layer haemorrhage, but it is identified within the ventricular cavity (Fig. 4B). Unlike the Levene[20] and Papile[21] classifications of intraventricular haemorrhage using cranial ultrasound and computed tomography, respectively, no classification using MRI has been devised. Cranial ultrasound is able to identify correctly the majority of intraventricular haemorrhage subsequently seen on MRI and has a strong positive predictive value. However, small haemorrhages are sometimes missed in the posterior horns of the lateral ventricles that may be identified as fluid levels on MRI.[2]

HAEMORRHAGIC PARENCHYMAL INFARCTION

Haemorrhagic parenchymal infarction is a lesion occurring within the white matter. It is usually adjacent to an intraventricular haemorrhage (Fig. 4C) and results from obstruction to venous drainage with subsequent white matter infarction. On T1-weighted sequences, acute haemorrhage is initially iso-intense and then becomes high-signal intensity; however, on T2-weighted sequences, the signal intensity of haemorrhage varies depending on the time between imaging and insult.[19] At term equivalent age, an haemorrhagic parenchymal infarction can often be seen as a cystic lesion in communication with the lateral ventricle. Care should be taken with non-communicating cysts as they can be mistaken for lesions due to periventricular leukomalacia if an haemorrhagic parenchymal infarction has not been previously identified. Prediction of hemiplegia in infants with a unilateral lesion depends upon the site of the haemorrhagic parenchymal infarction in relation to the trigone and any subsequent asymmetry of myelination within the posterior limb of the internal capsule.[22] This is not necessarily a result of direct damage to the posterior limb of the internal capsule, but due to secondary Wallerian degeneration.

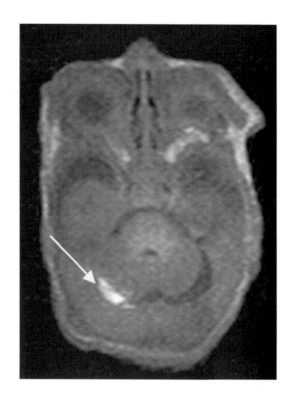

Fig. 5 T1-weighted axial image of a right-sided cerebellar haemorrhage (arrow) in an infant born at 25^{+4} weeks' gestational age and imaged at 26^{+6} weeks' gestational age.

CEREBELLAR HAEMORRHAGE

Cerebellar haemorrhage is a common finding during post mortem in preterm infants; however, it is not easily identified in the living preterm population using standard cranial ultrasound views. With the increasing use of brain MRI[23] and also cranial ultrasound through the posterior fontanelle,[24] cerebellar haemorrhage is being identified with greater frequency. On MRI, it is identified as high signal intensity on T1-weighted sequences (Fig. 5) and of variable signal intensity on T2-weighted sequences depending on the timing of imaging. A recent study has shown an incidence of about 9% on the first MRI after birth in a consecutive cohort of infants born at < 30 weeks' gestational age and imaged at a median age of 2 days.[23] Cerebellar haemorrhage tended to occur in the extremely preterm population born at < 26 weeks' gestational age and was often associated with an intraventricular haemorrhage. It was associated with a poor outcome, especially in infants with subsequent cerebellar atrophy. An association between cerebellar injury in the very low birth weight population and cerebral palsy has also been made.[25] Whether cerebellar haemorrhage influences the normal development of other structures within the brain, whether it is a marker of illness severity in these infants or whether it primarily influences outcome is an area for further investigation.

EXTRACEREBRAL HAEMORRHAGE

Extracerebral haemorrhage is not easily identified on cranial ultrasound unless it is large or associated with mid-line shift. MRI has greater sensitivity than

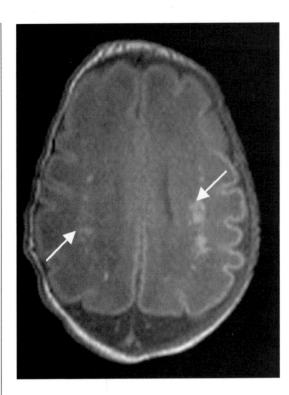

Fig. 6 T1-weighted axial image showing punctate white matter abnormalities at the level of the centrum semiovale in an infant born at 29^{+6} weeks' gestational age and imaged at 32^{+3} weeks' gestational age.

both cranial ultrasound and computed tomography in the identification of extracerebral haemorrhage.[26] Very little has been published concerning the incidence and outcome of these lesions in the preterm infant. Our own experience, in a consecutive cohort of infants born at < 30 weeks' gestational age and undergoing a brain MRI at a median age of 2 days, was an incidence of 5% and a normal developmental outcome in survivors without other significant intracranial pathology (unpublished data). The majority of haemorrhage was within the posterior fossa.

PUNCTATE WHITE MATTER ABNORMALITIES

Punctate abnormalities within the white matter in preterm infants are a common finding. They are seen as discrete areas of high-signal intensity on T1-weighted sequences (Fig. 6) and are less easily identified as low signal intensity lesions on T2-weighted sequences. They may represent haemorrhage; however, it is also possible that they represent small areas of infarction with capillary proliferation or areas of mineralisation. In infants born at < 30 weeks' gestational age, they can be identified on images taken soon after birth and are often still present at term equivalent age. Their persistence has also been noted on follow-up imaging at 2 years' corrected age when they are seen very clearly as areas of high-signal intensity on T2-weighted imaging. Their presence does not appear to be related to a short-term adverse neurodevelopmental outcome;[27] however, their persistence as focal abnormalities requires further investigation with neurodevelopmental assessments at later ages.

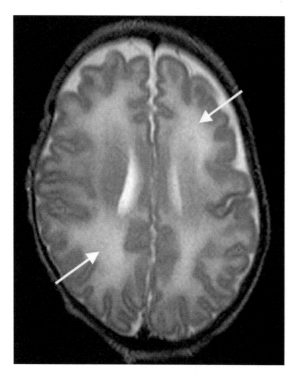

Fig. 7 T2-weighted axial image showing diffuse excessive high signal intensity in an infant born at 29 weeks' gestational age and imaged at term equivalent age.

DIFFUSE WHITE MATTER ABNORMALITIES

Diffuse excessive high-signal intensity (DEHSI) is an abnormality found throughout the white matter on T2-weighted imaging in about 75% of preterm infants when imaged at term equivalent age (Fig. 7).[11] It is not present on images of normal term born infants scanned at an equivalent gestational age. Its absence in normal term born infants and its high prevalence within the preterm population suggests that it either represents a process of abnormal development or one of subtle injury and it should not be assumed to represent mild periventricular leukomalacia. The histopathology underlying DEHSI remains uncertain as no postmortem correlates exist and there are no animal models published to date. However, indirect evidence of a pathological basis comes from diffusion weighted imaging studies as described in more detail later in this article.[28] Recent evidence suggests that DEHSI may be related to a poorer developmental outcome;[29] however, this needs to be further investigated in larger populations. A relationship with cerebral atrophy has also been proposed and this also needs to be further explored.[11]

PERIVENTRICULAR LEUKOMALACIA

Periventricular leukomalacia is a pathological diagnosis described histologically as 'softening of the white matter' due to ischaemia. On cranial ultrasound imaging, the initial stages of periventricular leukomalacia are represented by periventricular regions of increased echogenicity or 'flares'. More severe insults result in the development of white matter cysts. Cranial

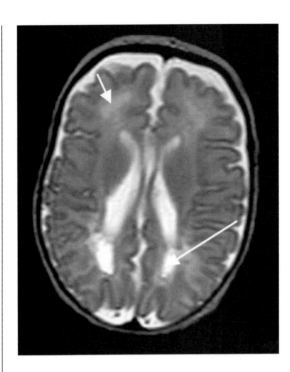

Fig. 8 T2-weighted axial image of periventricular leukomalacia with cysts in the posterior periventricular region (long arrow) and diffuse high signal abnormalities within the frontal white matter (short arrow) in an infant born at 30+5 weeks' gestational age and imaged at term equivalent age.

ultrasound demonstrates high reliability in the detection of cystic periventricular leukomalacia lesions[30] and the prediction of cerebral palsy,[6] but is less reliable in the detection of more subtle white matter injury. The severity of periventricular echogenicity on cranial ultrasound on early and later images has not been shown to correlate with white matter abnormalities on brain MRI in these infants.[7] On MRI, cystic lesions are the same signal intensity as CSF on both T1- and T2-weighted sequences (Fig. 8). MRI also provides additional information compared to cranial ultrasound, both at an early (within 4 weeks of birth) and a late (term equivalent age) time point.[31] Early MRI can identify a greater number of cysts and also the presence of associated punctate white matter lesions and basal ganglia lesions, but it remains to be shown that the identification of these lesions on MRI improves the prediction for motor deficits. MRI at term equivalent age may identify signal abnormalities within the posterior limb of the internal capsule that suggest abnormal myelination and provide a correlate for the development of cerebral palsy.[6] Diffusion weighted imaging has also been able to demonstrate more diffuse abnormalities of the white matter that are not apparent on conventional imaging in infants with cystic periventricular leukomalacia.[28]

The effect of periventricular leukomalacia on cerebral development has been investigated using quantitative MRI and tissue segmentation. Preterm infants with periventricular leukomalacia have decreased cortical grey matter, decreased myelinated white matter and an associated increase in CSF volume.[32] This suggests that early damage to periventricular white matter may have a significant impact on subsequent development of the cortical grey matter in the preterm infant.

CEREBRAL INFARCTION

This lesion, often referred to as a 'perinatal stroke', is more commonly seen in the term born population; however, it can also occur in the preterm infant and can be a postnatal insult. These lesions are rarely identified on cranial ultrasound in preterm infants within the first few days, but there is increasing echogenicity within the affected tissue during the first week after the insult. Subsequent cystic degeneration will often occur. In a series of 23 preterm infants studied using MRI by de Vries et al.,[33] the site of infarction was very variable. Infarction of the middle, anterior and posterior cerebral arteries was seen as well as insults involving lenticulostriate and cortical branches. Watershed infarctions can also occur. On MRI imaging these lesions are low-signal intensity on T1-weighted imaging and high-signal intensity on T2-weighted imaging within the appropriate arterial distribution or watershed area. In the term neonate, diffusion weighted imaging is able to identify cerebral infarction more clearly and at an earlier time point.[34] There are no studies published investigating diffusion weighted imaging in preterm cerebral infarction. The neurodevelopmental outcome of term infants with perinatal stoke is well documented using the pattern of injury affecting the basal ganglia, posterior limb of the internal capsule and the white matter.[35] If all three structures are affected then there is a high risk of hemiplegia; however, if only one or two of these structures are damaged the risk is much lower. Similar studies have not been conducted in preterm infants, but our experience suggests that the same principles apply.

BASAL GANGLIA AND THALAMIC INJURY

Basal ganglia and thalamic injury in the preterm infant can be haemorrhagic, ischaemic or metabolic in nature. Haemorrhage within the caudate head can occur due to secondary extension from a germinal layer haemorrhage and will be seen as high-signal intensity on T1-weighted imaging and initially as low-signal intensity on T2-weighted imaging. Large haemorrhages may show variable signal intensity on T2-weighted imaging depending on the timing of the scan. Hypoxic–ischaemic damage can also occur to these structures as in the term infant. However, in preterm infants, the thalamus appears to be more commonly affected than the basal ganglia.[36] The patterns of outcome for this type of injury are similar to that found for full-term infants. Hyper-bilirubinaemia is an uncommon, but potential, cause of basal ganglia injury and in critically ill infants the bilirubin level required to cause kernicterus may not be excessively high. A recent report has identified some abnormalities on ultrasound, but damage within the globus pallidus and subthalamic nuclei is best seen on MRI.[37] The optimal timing for MRI scanning in this condition is not fully evaluated.

INFECTION

Congenital cytomegalovirus, toxoplasmosis, rubella and herpes simplex can all potentially impact on the neonatal brain. Cranial ultrasound can detect cerebral abnormalities including calcification, lenticulostriate vasculopathy,

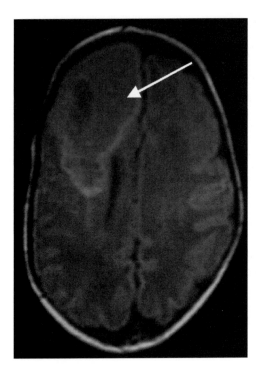

Fig. 9 T1-weighted axial image showing a right frontal abscess due to bacterial infection in an infant born at 34 weeks' gestational age and imaged at 37 weeks' gestational age.

periventricular cysts and ventricular dilatation. However, MRI is able to provide additional information especially concerning cerebral developmental abnormalities. A recent study by de Vries et al.[38] considered the MRI findings in preterm and term infants with congenital cytomegalovirus. Six infants were scanned during the neonatal period and they identified polymicrogyria in the perisylvian region, hippocampal dysplasia, cerebellar hypoplasia and also abnormalities of signal intensity in the white matter. Calcification was better seen on cranial ultrasound. There is a high incidence of neurological sequelae in infants with congenital infection and identification of underlying developmental abnormalities of the brain provides additional information for counselling parents about prognosis.

MRI also has a role in the imaging of infants with bacterial infection and it is important when suspecting infection to use a contrast agent such as gadolinium. Diffuse white matter injury related to episodes of hypoxia, ischaemia from hypotension, or damage from inflammatory cytokines can be identified using MRI, although echodensities will often be visible on cranial ultrasound. Abscesses can be missed on cranial ultrasound and when seen, MRI provides further information about their location and extent (Fig. 9). Sinus thrombosis can also occur in association with bacterial infection and this is difficult to identify on cranial ultrasound and requires brain MRI for diagnosis.

OTHER CEREBRAL ABNORMALITIES

Brain MRI has a role in the diagnosis and prognosis of a number of other disorders occurring in the preterm infant. Although uncommon, developmental abnormalities of the brain are often difficult to identify on cranial ultrasound,

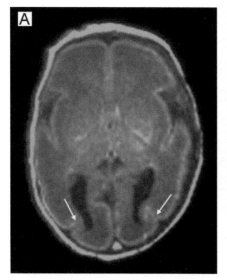 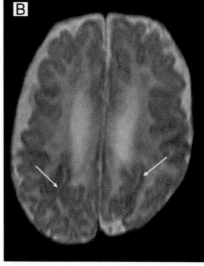

Fig. 10 T2-axial images showing a developmental abnormality of the posterior cortex with bilateral clefts in an infant born at 27^{+2} weeks' gestational age and imaged at (A) 31^{+1} weeks' gestational age and (B) 46^{+5} weeks' gestational age.

especially if they involve neuronal migration or cortical gyral abnormalities. MRI is able to identify these abnormalities with greater sensitivity (Fig. 10A,B). Developmental abnormalities of the brain are also associated with metabolic disorders. Hypoplasia or absence of the corpus callosum is well recognised in non-ketotic hyperglycinaemia and MR spectroscopy can identify increased levels of glycine within the brain. Impaired myelination, germinolytic cysts and abnormal cortical gyral patterns are cerebral features of perioxisomal disorders and several other metabolic disorders. Imaging of disorders affecting the brainstem and posterior fossa, such as ponto-cerebellar hypoplasia, Dandy Walker malformations and posterior fossa tumours, relies on MRI for optimal identification and classification.

OTHER MRI TECHNIQUES

DIFFUSION WEIGHTED AND DIFFUSION TENSOR IMAGING

Diffusion weighted imaging demonstrates the molecular motion of water within tissues. Apparent diffusion coefficients can be calculated and provide a quantification of this motion in units of mm^2/s. Diffusion weighted imaging can be used to investigate normal cerebral development and also cerebral injury in infants born prematurely. Diffusion decreases with increasing gestational age as the water content of the brain diminishes. Periventricular leukomalacia has been investigated using diffusion weighted imaging and abnormalities within the white matter can be detected before cystic lesions develop.[39] Increased diffusion has also been identified within the white matter of infants with DEHSI.[28] Apparent diffusion coefficient values are significantly higher in DEHSI than in infants with normal appearing white matter, but do

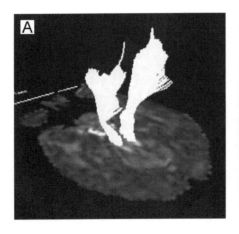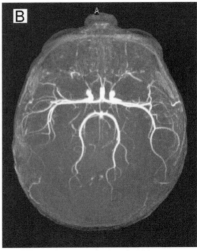

Fig. 11 (A) Tractography. An axial slice from an infant born at 28 weeks' gestational age and imaged at 44 weeks' gestational age showing corticospinal tracts superimposed on the diffusion tensor image. (B) Magnetic resonance angiogram of the intracranial vessels of an infant born at 30 weeks' gestational age and scanned at term equivalent age.

not differ significantly from those in infants with white matter abnormalities. Diffusion weighted imaging has, therefore, provided indirect quantitative evidence that DEHSI has an underlying pathological basis.

Diffusion tensor imaging measures the directional dependence of water motion in a restricted environment, known as anisotropy. Even before myelination occurs, diffusion of water is relatively free in the direction of the white matter fibre tracts and relatively restricted in any other direction. This directional diffusion within white matter tracts increases with increasing gestational age.[40] Tractography is an extension of diffusion tensor imaging that identifies the direction of maximum diffusion within a structure containing fibre tracts, allowing the course of the fibre tracts to be defined (Fig. 11A).

VOLUMETRIC TECHNIQUES

A number of studies have used computational morphometric techniques to investigate the structural effects of preterm birth on brain development in older children who were born preterm. A comprehensive review of this literature is beyond the scope of this article as we have focused on MRI up to term equivalent age. One newer computer-based volumetric technique being used on early images is deformation based morphometry. This technique warps 3-D brain volumes into a common reference space and statistical information about local volume change is extracted. This computational morphometric approach has been used to quantify structural differences between the preterm brain at term equivalent age and the term born brain.[41] One advantage over other volumetric techniques is that it does not require prior tissue segmentation.

Table 2 Information provided on neurodevelopmental outcome by brain MRI at term equivalent age

Lesion	MRI abnormality	Outcome
Haemorrhagic parenchymal infarction	Asymmetry of myelination within the posterior limb of the internal capsule	Hemiplegia[22]
Cystic periventricular leukomalacia	Delayed/abnormal myelination within the posterior limb of the internal capsule	Spastic diplegia/quadriplegia depending on severity[31]
Focal white matter injury	Punctate white matter lesions	Normal developmental outcome[27]*
Diffuse white matter injury	Diffuse excessive high-signal intensity	Decreased developmental quotient at 2 years' corrected age[29]*
Cerebral infarction	Abnormality of the basal ganglia, posterior limb of the internal capsule and cerebral hemisphere (3/3 structures)	Hemiplegia[35]*
Hypoxic–ischaemic basal ganglia, thalamic and brainstem injury	Abnormal signal in the posterior lentiform, thalamic nuclei and brainstem	Spastic quadriplegia, severe bulbar difficulties and low IQ
Cerebellar haemorrhage	Cerebellar haemorrhage with subsequent cerebellar atrophy	Increased risk of cerebral palsy and low IQ[23]*
Extracerebral haemorrhage	Isolated extracerebral haemorrhage	Normal developmental outcome*

*Indicates that this is the current knowledge about these lesions and that studies are on-going.

MAGNETIC RESONANCE ANGIOGRAPHY

MR angiography is well established in adult medicine, but appropriate scanning parameters are currently being identified for neonates (Fig. 11B). Venography has been primarily used to visualise vein of Galen aneurysms in neonates; however, angiography in the preterm infant can now be used to define normal variations of cerebral vasculature and abnormalities relating to haemorrhage and thrombosis. The advantage of MR angiography is that it is non-invasive and contrast medium is not required.

Key points for clinical practice

- MRI does not replace cranial ultrasound as a technique for imaging the preterm brain; it is complementary and can provide additional information.

- MRI can be performed safely in infants as immature as 23 weeks' gestation, but experienced and skilled staff are required.

- The most useful timing for a single MRI examination to be performed in the preterm infant is at term equivalent age and important information about prognosis can be gathered from this image (see Table 2).

- The majority of neurodevelopmental problems in preterm infants probably relate to subtle injury or abnormalities of cerebral development rather than focal lesions.

- Newer MRI techniques of diffusion weighted imaging, tractography and deformation based morphometry will increase our understanding of the effects of injury on brain development in the preterm infant.

References

1. Foulder-Hughes LA,.Cooke RW. Motor, cognitive, and behavioural disorders in children born very preterm. *Dev Med Child Neurol* 2003; **45**: 97–103.
2. Maalouf EF, Duggan PJ, Counsell SJ *et al*. Comparison of findings on cranial ultrasound and magnetic resonance imaging in preterm infants. *Pediatrics* 2001; **107**: 719–727.
3. Larroque B, Marret S, Ancel PY *et al*. White matter damage and intraventricular hemorrhage in very preterm infants: the EPIPAGE study. *J Pediatr* 2003; **143**: 477–483.
4. Abernethy LJ, Palaniappan M, Cooke RW. Quantitative magnetic resonance imaging of the brain in survivors of very low birth weight. *Arch Dis Child* 2002; **87**: 279–283.
5. Jongmans M, Mercuri E, de Vries L, Dubowitz L, Henderson SE. Minor neurological signs and perceptual-motor difficulties in prematurely born children. *Arch Dis Child* 1997; **76**: F9–F14.
6. De Vries LS, Van Haastert IL, Rademaker KJ, Koopman C, Groenendaal F. Ultrasound abnormalities preceding cerebral palsy in high-risk preterm infants. *J Pediatr* 2004; **144**: 815–820.
7. Miller SP, Cozzio CC, Goldstein RB *et al*. Comparing the diagnosis of white matter injury in premature newborns with serial MR imaging and transfontanel ultrasonography findings. *AJNR Am J Neuroradiol* 2003; **24**: 1661–1669.

8. Battin M, Maalouf EF, Counsell S *et al*. Physiological stability of preterm infants during magnetic resonance imaging. *Early Hum Dev* 1998; **52**: 101–110.
9. Ajayi-Obe M, Saeed N, Cowan FM, Rutherford MA, Edwards AD. Reduced development of cerebral cortex in extremely preterm infants. *Lancet* 2000; **356**: 1162–1163.
10. Huppi PS, Warfield S, Kikinis R *et al*. Quantitative magnetic resonance imaging of brain development in premature and mature newborns. *Ann Neurol* 1998; **43**: 224–235.
11. Maalouf EF, Duggan PJ, Rutherford MA *et al*. Magnetic resonance imaging of the brain in a cohort of extremely preterm infants. *J Pediatr* 1999; **135**: 351–357.
12. Felderhoff-Mueser U, Rutherford MA, Squier WV *et al*. Relationship between MR imaging and histopathologic findings of the brain in extremely sick preterm infants. *AJNR Am J Neuroradiol* 1999; **20**: 1349–1357.
13. Counsell SJ, Maalouf EF, Fletcher AM *et al*. MR imaging assessment of myelination in the very preterm brain. *AJNR Am J Neuroradiol* 2002; **23**: 872–881.
14. van de Bor M, Guit GL, Schreuder AM *et al*. Does very preterm birth impair myelination of the central nervous system? *Neuropediatrics* 1990; **21**: 37–39.
15. Guit GL, van de Bor M, den Ouden L, Wondergem JH. Prediction of neurodevelopmental outcome in the preterm infant: MR-staged myelination compared with cranial US. *Radiology* 1990; **175**: 107–109.
16. McArdle CB, Richardson CJ, Nicholas DA *et al*. Developmental features of the neonatal brain: MR imaging. Part II. Ventricular size and extracerebral space. *Radiology* 1987; **162**: 230–234.
17. Battin M, Rutherford MA. MRI of the brain in preterm infants: 24 weeks' gestation to term. In: Rutherford M (ed) *MRI of the Neonatal Brain*. London: W.B. Saunders, 2002; 25–49.
18. Battin MR, Maalouf EF, Counsell SJ *et al*. Magnetic resonance imaging of the brain in very preterm infants: visualization of the germinal matrix, early myelination, and cortical folding. *Pediatrics* 1998; **101**: 957–962.
19. Rutherford MA. Hemorrhagic lesions of the newborn brain. In: Rutherford M (ed) *MRI of the Neonatal Brain*. London: W.B. Saunders, 2002; 172–200.
20. Levene MI, de Crespigny LC. Classification of intraventricular hemorrhage. *Lancet* 1983; **1**: 643.
21. Papile LA, Burstein J, Burstein R, Koffler H. Incidence and evolution of subependymal and intraventricular hemorrhage: a study of infants with birth weights less than 1,500 gm. *J Pediatr* 1978; **92**: 529–534.
22. De Vries LS, Roelants-Van Rijn AM, Rademaker KJ *et al*. Unilateral parenchymal haemorrhagic infarction in the preterm infant. *Eur J Paediatr Neurol* 2001; **5**: 139–149.
23. Dyet L, Kennea NL, Counsell S *et al*. Cerebellar haemorrhage and neurodevelopmental outcome in a cohort of preterm infants. *Pediatr Res* 2004; **55**: 416A.
24. Merrill JD, Piecuch RE, Fell SC, Barkovich AJ, Goldstein RB. A new pattern of cerebellar hemorrhages in preterm infants. *Pediatrics* 1998; **102**: E62.
25. Johnsen SD, Tarby TJ, Lewis KS, Bird R, Prenger E. Cerebellar infarction: an unrecognized complication of very low birthweight. *J Child Neurol* 2002; **17**: 320–324.
26. Keeney SE, Adcock EW, McArdle CB. Prospective observations of 100 high-risk neonates by high-field (1.5 Tesla) magnetic resonance imaging of the central nervous system: I. Intraventricular and extracerebral lesions. *Pediatrics* 1991; **87**: 421–430.
27. Cornette LG, Tanner SF, Ramenghi LA *et al*. Magnetic resonance imaging of the infant brain: anatomical characteristics and clinical significance of punctate lesions. *Arch Dis Child* 2002; **86**: F171–F177.
28. Counsell SJ, Allsop JM, Harrison MC *et al*. Diffusion-weighted imaging of the brain in preterm infants with focal and diffuse white matter abnormality. *Pediatrics* 2003; **112**: 1–7.
29. Dyet L, Kennea NL, Counsell S *et al*. Diffuse white matter abnormalities on magnetic resonance imaging of the brain in preterm infants and neurodevelopmental outcome. *Pediatr Res* 2004; **55**: 424A.
30. Inder TE, Anderson NJ, Spencer C, Wells S, Volpe JJ. White matter injury in the premature infant: a comparison between serial cranial sonographic and MR findings at term. *AJNR Am J Neuroradiol* 2003; **24**: 805–809.
31. Roelants-Van Rijn AM, Groenendaal F, Beek FJ *et al*. Parenchymal brain injury in the preterm infant: comparison of cranial ultrasound, MRI and neurodevelopmental

outcome. *Neuropediatrics* 2001; **32**: 80–89.

32. Inder TE, Huppi PS, Warfield S *et al.* Periventricular white matter injury in the premature infant is followed by reduced cerebral cortical gray matter volume at term. *Ann Neurol* 1999; **46**: 755–760.

33. De Vries LS, Groenendaal F, Meiners LC. Ischaemic lesions in the preterm brain. In: Rutherford M (ed) *MRI of the Neonatal Brain*. London: W.B. Saunders, 2002; 155–169.

34. Cowan FM, Pennock JM, Hanrahan JD, Manji KP, Edwards AD. Early detection of cerebral infarction and hypoxic ischemic encephalopathy in neonates using diffusion-weighted magnetic resonance imaging. *Neuropediatrics* 1994; **25**: 172–175.

35. Mercuri E, Rutherford M, Cowan F *et al.* Early prognostic indicators of outcome in infants with neonatal cerebral infarction: a clinical, electroencephalogram, and magnetic resonance imaging study. *Pediatrics* 1999; **103**: 39–46.

36. Barkovich AJ, Sargent SK. Profound asphyxia in the premature infant: imaging findings. *AJNR Am J Neuroradiol* 1995; **16**: 1837–1846.

37. Govaert P, Lequin M, Swarte R *et al.* Changes in globus pallidus with (pre)term kernicterus. *Pediatrics* 2003; **112**: 1256–1263.

38. De Vries LS, Gunardi H, Barth PG *et al.* The spectrum of cranial ultrasound and magnetic resonance imaging abnormalities in congenital cytomegalovirus infection. *Neuropediatrics* 2004; **35**: 113–119.

39. Inder T, Huppi PS, Zientara GP *et al.* Early detection of periventricular leukomalacia by diffusion-weighted magnetic resonance imaging techniques. *J Pediatr* 1999; **134**: 631–634.

40. Partridge SC, Mukherjee P, Henry RG *et al.* Diffusion tensor imaging: serial quantitation of white matter tract maturity in premature newborns. *Neuroimage* 2004; **22**: 1302–1314.

41. Boardman J, Bhatia K, Counsell S. An evaluation of deformation-based morphometry applied to the developing human brain and detection of volumetric changes associated with preterm birth. *Lecture Notes in Computer Science* 2003; **2878**: 697–704.

Oliver Tunstall-Pedoe Irene Roberts

8

Neonatal thrombocytopenia

Thrombocytopenia is a common clinical problem in neonatal units, occurring in around one-third of babies requiring intensive care. Although platelet counts in the fetus have reached normal levels by as early as 16 weeks' gestation, differences between neonatal and adult megakaryopoiesis predispose neonates to the development of thrombocytopenia. Most textbooks quote a long and complicated list of causes of neonatal thrombocytopenia, many of which are extremely rare. However, the natural history of the condition often takes one of a small number of patterns which helps to identify the more likely causes in the majority of babies. Recognition of these patterns, along with an understanding of the mechanisms involved, can help neonatologists and haematologists to identify quickly those babies in need of urgent intervention and to plan appropriate and focused investigations.

This chapter reviews current knowledge of the causes and mechanisms of neonatal thrombocytopenia to provide the clinician with a structured approach to the investigation, diagnosis and management of this common clinical condition.

MEGAKARYOPOIESIS AND PLATELET PRODUCTION IN THE FETUS AND NEONATE

ONTOGENY OF MEGAKARYOPOIESIS

Haemopoiesis in humans first occurs in the yolk sac in the third week of gestation; at this stage, the majority of blood cells produced are erythrocytes.[1]

Oliver Tunstall-Pedoe MB BChir BAHons MRCPCH
Clinical Research Fellow and Haematology Specialist Registrar, Department of Haematology,
Hammersmith Hospital, Du Cane Road, London W12 0NN, UK. E-mail: o.tunstallpedoe@imperial.ac.uk

Irene Roberts MD FRCP FRCPath DRCOG (for correspondence)
Professor of Paediatric Haematology, Department of Haematology, Hammersmith Hospital, Du
Cane Road, London W12 0NN, UK. E-mail: irene.roberts@imperial.ac.uk

By 5 weeks' gestation, when the main site of haemopoiesis changes to the aorto-gonad-mesonephros region of the dorsal aorta, megakaryocyte progenitor cells start to be produced.[1] Soon afterwards, aorto-gonad-mesonephros-derived haemopoietic stem cells migrate to the liver which, by 6–8 weeks' gestation, becomes the primary site of blood cell production, including megakaryopoiesis, for the remaining months of fetal life.[1,2] Platelets first appear in the circulation at 5–6 weeks' post-conceptual age.[2] The platelet count rises steadily with an overall mean count of $159 \pm 34 \times 10^9/l$ by 10–17 weeks' gestation and $240 \pm 60 \times 10^9/l$ at 18 weeks' gestation,[2,3] remaining constant thereafter until birth and beyond.[2,4] Therefore, the lower limit of normal for the platelet count for all neonates, regardless of gestational age, is the same as in older children and adults (*i.e.* $> 150 \times 10^9/l$).

REGULATION OF MEGAKARYOPOIESIS AND PLATELET PRODUCTION

Thrombopoietin, the main regulator of platelet homeostasis in humans, is believed to have a similar function in the fetus and neonate.[5,6] Thrombopoietin mRNA has been detected from 6 weeks' post conception and is produced mainly by the liver.[7] Most healthy newborns have detectable circulating thrombopoietin, and increased thrombopoietin levels have been found in neonates with thrombocytopenia due to reduced megakaryopoiesis and/or platelet production.[8,9] Indeed, there is a negative correlation between circulating thrombopoietin levels and megakaryocyte mass, suggesting that receptor binding and metabolism of thrombopoietin are the main regulators of thrombopoietin levels, as in adult platelet homeostasis.[5] Mouse models show that expression of the genes for both thrombopoietin (*Tpo*) and its receptor (*c-mpl*) are important for megakaryopoiesis since knockout mice for both genes are severely thrombocytopenic with 10–15% of the normal platelet level.[10] Similarly, the megakaryocyte transcription factor GATA1 has been shown to be essential for megakaryocyte differentiation and mutation of GATA1 has recently been shown to cause severe abnormalities of neonatal megakaryopoiesis (see below).[11]

PREDISPOSITION TO THROMBOCYTOPENIA IN PRETERM NEONATES

Although the healthy fetus and neonate can generate and maintain platelet counts at adult levels from early in gestation, there is increasing evidence of differences in fetal and neonatal megakaryopoiesis which predispose the sick neonate to thrombocytopenia. First, in the normal fetus, megakaryocytes isolated from the liver and bone marrow are significantly smaller and more immature than those found in adult bone marrow and, therefore, have a reduced ability to make platelets.[3,12] This may be because immature megakaryocyte progenitors have recently been shown to be less sensitive to thrombopoietin than progenitors which have completed their proliferative programme.[13] Second, both preterm and term neonates appear to have a reduced ability to produce large amounts of thrombopoietin in response to thrombocytopenia.[7,8] Finally, many babies with early thrombocytopenia have reduced numbers of megakaryocyte progenitors.[14]

INCIDENCE OF THROMBOCYTOPENIA IN NEONATES

The incidence of neonatal thrombocytopenia has been investigated by many groups and varies considerably depending on the population studied. Cross-sectional studies of thrombocytopenia at birth have shown a range of 0.5–4.1% of neonates with a platelet count of $< 150 \times 10^9/l$.[15–17] Burrows and Kelton[15] studied cord blood from 1350 unselected newborns and found an incidence of 4.1%. More recently, in a study[16] of term neonates born to native Finnish women in Helsinki, 89/4489 (2%) were found to have a platelet count $< 150 \times 10^9/l$; in an even larger study of 8388 newborns, thrombocytopenia was recorded in 0.5% of cases.[17] What is probably more important is the availability

Table 1 Causes of neonatal thrombocytopenia

Placental insufficiency
      Maternal hypertension and/or pre-eclampsia
      Intrauterine growth restriction
      Maternal diabetes

Immune
      Alloimmune
      Autoimmune (maternal autoimmune thrombocytopenia)
      Neonatal lupus

Infection
      Congenital: cytomegalovirus, *Toxoplasma*, rubella, HIV, Coxsackie
      Perinatal: Group B streptococci, *Haemophilus influenzae*, *E. coli*

Congenital/inherited
      Aneuploidy: trisomies 13, 18 and 21; triploidy
      Bone marrow failure affecting megakaryocytes (*e.g.* congenital amegakaryocytic thrombocytopenia, thrombocytopenia absent radius syndrome)
      Bone marrow failure syndromes with pancytopenia (*e.g.* Fanconi anaemia)
      Myelodysplasia (*e.g.* monosomy 7)
      Immunodeficiencies (*e.g.* Wiskott Aldrich, haemophagocytic lymphohistiocytosis)
      Platelet function disorders with thrombocytopenia (*e.g.* Bernard Soulier syndrome)

Disseminated intravascular coagulation
      Perinatal asphyxia (and whole body cooling)
      Bacterial infection
      Congenital thrombotic thrombocytopenic purpura (ADAMTS-13 deficiency)

Other
      Thrombosis – aortic, renal
      Kasabach Merritt
      Hepatic haemangioendothelioma
      Metabolic – propionic acidaemia, methylmalonic acidaemia
      Congenital leukaemia
      Heparin-induced thrombocytopenia
      Subcutaneous fat necrosis of the newborn
      Exchange transfusion
      Rhesus haemolytic disease of the newborn

of information about the incidence of thrombocytopenia in those babies most at risk (sick and preterm neonates) and the incidence of severe thrombocytopenia (platelets < 50 x 10^9/l).

Several studies have shown that the incidence of thrombocytopenia is much higher in sick and preterm neonates: around one-third of all babies admitted to neonatal units will be thrombocytopenic (platelets < 150 x 10^9/l) during their admission[18,19] and around 10% will have a platelet count of < 100 x 10^9/l.[20] Fortunately, the majority of episodes of neonatal thrombocytopenia are moderate or mild and are not associated with clinical sequelae.[17,19,21] However, around 20% of episodes of thrombocytopenia in neonatal intensive care unit patients are severe (platelets < 50 x 10^9/l)[17,19] and a number of studies have shown that these babies are at increased risk of haemorrhage.[19,21,22]

CAUSES OF THROMBOCYTOPENIA

A comprehensive list of the causes of neonatal thrombocytopenia is shown in Table 1. Such a list is useful for identifying rare causes of thrombocytopenia. However, most cases are due to common disorders and a more practical classification of neonatal thrombocytopenia is based on the age of the baby at the time the thrombocytopenia develops. The timing of the onset of thrombocytopenia, together with associated clinical features, can be used to identify the cause of the vast majority of cases of neonatal thrombocytopenia.[23]

There are two main patterns of neonatal thrombocytopenia based on the time of presentation: (i) early-onset neonatal thrombocytopenia (presenting before 72 h of age) which almost always has its origin in fetal life; and (ii) late-onset neonatal thrombocytopenia (presenting after 72 h of age) which is usually secondary to post-natal events.[23]

EARLY-ONSET NEONATAL THROMBOCYTOPENIA

Early thrombocytopenia constitutes 75% of all neonatal thrombocytopenia (Table 2). Babies may present at birth or during the first 72 h of life.[14,24] The majority of cases are in preterm neonates born following pregnancies

Table 2 Most common causes of early neonatal thrombocytopenia

Placental insufficiency	
	Maternal hypertension and/or pre-eclampsia
	Intra-uterine growth restriction
	Maternal diabetes
Immune	
	Alloimmune
	Autoimmune (maternal autoimmune thrombocytopenia)
Infection	
	Congenital: cytomegalovirus, *Toxoplasma*
	Perinatal: Group B streptococci, *H. influenzae, E. coli*
Congenital/inherited	
	Aneuploidy: trisomies 13, 18 and 21
Disseminated intravascular coagulation	
	Perinatal asphyxia

complicated by placental insufficiency and/or fetal hypoxia e.g. maternal pre-eclampsia, fetal intra-uterine growth restriction, or, less commonly, maternal diabetes mellitus.[23] Such babies have characteristic haematological features which are not difficult to recognise (see below). They usually have a platelet count of 100–200 x 10^9/l at birth, falling to a nadir of 50–100 x 10^9/l at days 4–5 of life before recovering to normal by 7–10 days of life; the platelet count does not usually fall below 50 x 10^9/l.[24] Conversely, early neonatal thrombocytopenias which do not conform to the above pattern are likely to be a marker of significant pathology and may require specific management. Causes include congenital infection, bacterial sepsis, aneuploidy, immune causes and congenital/inherited thrombocytopenias. Early-onset thrombocytopenias which persist for more than 7–10 days are also unusual and warrant further investigation. As most other forms of thrombocytopenia will have resolved by this time, the likely causes of prolonged thrombocytopenia are: immune, congenital infections, and congenital/inherited thrombocytopenias.

LATE-ONSET NEONATAL THROMBOCYTOPENIA (> 72 H OF AGE)

Late-onset thrombocytopenia in neonatal intensive care unit patients is usually caused by sepsis or necrotising enterocolitis.[19] It has a distinctly different pattern to that seen in early-onset thrombocytopenia associated with placental insufficiency.[23] Isolated thrombocytopenia may be the first sign of sepsis or necrotising enterocolitis but, more commonly, thrombocytopenia manifests at the same time as the early signs of these conditions. Our group recently retrospectively reviewed all cases of severe thrombocytopenia occurring in our neonatal intensive care unit over a period of 3 years to assess the clinical associations, therapy and outcome of neonates.[19] There were 901 admissions of which 53 (6%) developed at least one episode of severe thrombocytopenia. The majority 44/53 (83%) of these neonates were preterm and late-onset sepsis was the commonest clinical condition occurring in association with severe thrombocytopenia: 34/44 (77%) had evidence of sepsis and 5 neonates (11%) developed severe thrombocytopenia during necrotising enterocolitis.

CONDITIONS LEADING TO CLINICALLY SIGNIFICANT NEONATAL THROMBOCYTOPENIA

IMMUNE CAUSES OF SEVERE NEONATAL THROMBOCYTOPENIA

Amongst the most clinically important causes of thrombocytopenia in the newborn are immune diseases. Although relatively uncommon, they can affect otherwise normal term infants with potentially devastating effects. They are caused by maternal IgG allo- or auto-antibodies crossing the placenta and destroying fetal platelets and megakaryocytes. Affected babies often develop severe thrombocytopenia and are at increased risk of intracranial haemorrhage and death.

Neonatal allo-immune thrombocytopenia
Neonatal alloimmune thrombocytopenia is the platelet equivalent of the haemolytic disease of the newborn. Like haemolytic disease of the newborn, it is caused by maternal sensitisation to fetal antigens inherited from the father.

In contrast to haemolytic disease of the newborn, it is seen in the first pregnancy in 50% of cases (reviewed by Kaplan[25]). Maternal anti-platelet antibodies are detectable in 1/350 pregnancies and neonatal alloimmune thrombocytopenia occurs in 1/1000 live births though it is thought that around 25% of cases are clinically silent.[25–27] In Caucasians, antibodies are most commonly directed against HPA-1a (80%), HPA-5b (10–15%) and occasionally anti-HPA-3a and anti-HPA-1b.[25–27] In Asian populations, antibodies are more commonly directed against HPA-4.[25] The development of antibodies against HPA-1a in HPA-1a-negative women is strongly associated with HLA DRB3 0101 (odds ratio 140).[27]

Neonatal alloimmune thrombocytopenia usually presents in otherwise well, term neonates with unexplained bruising and purpura. The platelet count is usually < 30 x 10^9/l. Up to 20% of affected infants will suffer serious bleeding including intracranial haemorrhage. This occurs *in utero* in 25–50% of cases and is associated with long-term neurodevelopmental sequelae in 20% of survivors (reviewed by Roberts and Murray[23] and Kaplan[25]).

Laboratory diagnosis is made by demonstrating anti-platelet antibodies (usually HPA-1a) in maternal serum which are directed against paternal antigens. This is done using indirect immunofluorescence testing and the monoclonal antibody (specific) immobilisation of platelet antigens.[17,25] Platelet genotypes of the parents and baby determined by PCR are available as confirmatory tests in reference laboratories.[25]

Treatment of mildly affected babies (platelets > 50 x 10^9/l and no evidence of intracranial or other significant haemorrhage) is not required although the platelet count should be monitored for the first 5 days after delivery as it usually falls over this time.[23,25,28] There is also no evidence that treatment of moderately affected infants (platelets 30–50 x 10^9/l) is necessary unless they have any evidence of bleeding.[28] By contrast, severely affected infants with neonatal alloimmune thrombocytopenia (platelets < 30 x 10^9/l and/or evidence of intracranial or other major bleeding) should be promptly transfused with HPA-compatible platelets.[25,28] In 95% of cases, HPA-1a negative, HPA-5b negative platelets are suitable. In the UK, there is a pool of suitable donors and these platelets are available at short notice from the National Blood Service; washed maternal platelets are virtually never indicated.[28] The results of serological investigations are not necessary before commencement of treatment. If severe thrombocytopenia and/or haemorrhage persists despite HPA-compatible platelets, intravenous IgG (total dose 2 g/kg over 2–5 days) is often useful in ameliorating the thrombocytopenia until spontaneous recovery occurs 1–6 weeks after birth.[23,25]

The risk of recurrence of neonatal alloimmune thrombocytopenia in subsequent pregnancies is high, approaching 100% where the father is homozygous for the incompatible platelet antigen. Management of such 'at-risk' pregnancies is controversial (reviewed by Roberts and Murray[23]). The principal options are an invasive approach using fetal blood sampling plus fetal transfusion with HPA-compatible platelets if thrombocytopenia is detected or a non-invasive approach relying on maternal intravenous IgG therapy; each approach has evidence to support it.[23]

Maternal autoimmune thrombocytopenia

Maternal platelet auto-antibodies occur in 1–2:1000 pregnancies.[17,23,29] However, neonatal thrombocytopenia due to transplacental passage of maternal auto-antibodies is much less of a clinical problem in maternal autoimmune thrombocytopenia than in neonatal alloimmune thrombocytopenia. This is because significant thrombocytopenia only occurs in 10% of neonates, intracranial haemorrhage in 1% or less (reviewed by Kelton[29]) and fetal loss in around 1%.[30] Fetal blood sampling and/or Caesarean delivery in mothers with maternal autoimmune thrombocytopenia are, therefore, no longer regarded as necessary, irrespective of the maternal platelet count during pregnancy.[29] The most useful predictors of significant fetal or neonatal thrombocytopenia are the severity of the maternal autoimmune thrombocytopenia and/or platelet count during pregnancy and the occurrence of severe thrombocytopenia in a previous neonate.[29,30]

All neonates of mothers with autoimmune thrombocytopenia should have their platelet count checked at birth.[23,29] There are no additional useful diagnostic laboratory tests. Platelet counts are at their lowest after 2–3 days and a repeat count at this time is recommended in all thrombocytopenic infants.[23] The platelet count will typically rise after about 7 days but, as in neonatal alloimmune thrombocytopenia, in a small number of cases thrombocytopenia persists for several weeks. Neonates with severe thrombocytopenia (platelets < 30 x 109/l) usually respond promptly to treatment with intravenous immunoglobulin (total dose 2 g/kg over 2–5 days).[29]

NEONATAL THROMBOCYTOPENIA DUE TO INFECTION

Late onset sepsis and necrotising enterocolitis

Bacterial sepsis and/or necrotising enterocolitis are the most frequent causes of severe thrombocytopenia ($< 50 \times 10^9/l$) in neonates and the most common cause of late-onset thrombocytopenia.[19] In a cohort of 39 neonates with severe thrombocytopenia associated with sepsis and/or necrotising enterocolitis, thrombocytopenia developed at a median post-natal age of 8 days (range, 1–37 days) and in over 75% of cases the platelet count dropped precipitously, from normal to below $50 \times 10^9/L$, within 48 h.[19] Severe thrombocytopenia was prolonged, the platelet count taking a median of 8 days (range, 2–50 days) to rise again consistently above $50 \times 10^9/l$. Evidence of disseminated intravascular coagulation was seen in fewer than 10% of neonates confirming previous studies indicating that this is not a frequent occurrence in this setting. Significant haemorrhage (*e.g.* intraventricular haemorrhage grades 3–4) was common, occurring in 7/44 of the preterm neonates (16%), although the initial bleeding episode had almost invariably occurred prior to the development of severe thrombocytopenia.[19] Five of the 44 preterm neonates with severe thrombocytopenia died prior to discharge: all 5 had a platelet nadir $< 30 \times 10^9/l$ and all had received platelet transfusions.[19]

A number of lines of evidence now indicate that impaired platelet production is an important component of the marked thrombocytopenia seen in association with neonatal sepsis and necrotising enterocolitis. Thrombocytopenia often persists long after these conditions have been controlled, suggesting that on-going platelet consumption is unlikely to be the reason for the continued low platelet count.[19] Also, a number of groups have reported raised thrombopoietin levels in septic neonates with thrombocytopenia, consistent with impairment of megakaryopoiesis and platelet production.[9,31,32] Our group has also shown lower numbers of circulating megakaryocyte progenitor cells in preterm neonates with sepsis-associated thrombocytopenia when compared to septic controls who maintained normal platelet counts.[32] Together, these findings suggest that platelet production is compromised in sepsis/necrotising enterocolitis although the mechanism for this remains to be explained.

Perinatal infection

Perinatal bacterial infection occurs in 1–2:1000 newborns as a whole and in up to 2% of very low birth weight neonates. The commonest organisms are group B streptococci and *Escherichia coli*. A recent study showed that thrombocytopenia develops in about 50% of such cases.[33] In contrast to late-onset neonatal sepsis, disseminated intravascular coagulation is an important mechanism of thrombocytopenia probably because of the severity of the sepsis syndrome induced by the causative organisms and the fact that infection has often begun prior to delivery before effective treatment can be instituted.

Congenital viral and Toxoplasma infections

Thrombocytopenia is a common finding in congenital viral or *Toxoplasma* infections. It is usually present in combination with other features suggestive of congenital infection, *e.g.* intracranial calcification, hepatosplenomegaly, jaundice or reactive lymphocytes. The most common congenital infection causing thrombocytopenia is that due to cytomegalovirus. Maternal cytomegalovirus infection during pregnancy results in congenital infection in about 0.5–1% of all newborns.[34] Only 10–15% of such infants have symptomatic disease but up to 75% of these will have significant thrombocytopenia (platelets < 100 x 10^9/l).[34] There is often accompanying neutropenia which, as with the thrombocytopenia, can sometimes persist for several months.

The other main virally-induced neonatal thrombocytopenias are due to rubella, HIV and Coxsackie infections, although congenital rubella is now very rare in countries with a comprehensive immunisation programme. The mechanism of virus-associated congenital thrombocytopenia is unclear; however, recent reports suggest that, at least in the case of cytomegalovirus, viruses can directly infect and inhibit megakaryocytes and their precursors resulting in impaired platelet production. Congenital toxoplasmosis affects 1:2000–3000 newborns, depending on geographical location and dietary practices, and is associated with thrombocytopenia in around 40% of affected neonates.[35]

CONGENITAL AND INHERITED THROMBOCYTOPENIAS

Inherited thrombocytopenias

Although these disorders are rare, they give important insight into megakaryopoiesis. The genetic basis for many of these disorders has recently been identified: defects in *c-mpl*, the thrombopoietin receptor, cause congenital amegakaryocytic thrombocytopenia; mutations in *RUNX1(AML1)* give rise to the familial platelet syndrome with predisposition to acute myeloid leukaemia; mutations in another transcription factor, GATA-1, cause the syndrome X-linked thrombocytopenia with dyserythropoiesis; and mutations in the myosin heavy chain A gene, *MYH9*, cause a variety of different rare giant platelet syndromes, including the May-Hegglin anomaly.[11,36] In most cases, the thrombocytopenia is due to reduced platelet production secondary to abnormal haemopoietic stem cell development and in most neonates, but not all, there are associated congenital anomalies which are useful in guiding investigations and establishing the diagnosis.

In some disorders, such as Bernard-Soulier syndrome and Wiskott-Aldrich syndrome, platelet function is also abnormal, although bleeding is not usually severe in the neonatal period. Wiskott-Aldrich syndrome and X-linked thrombocytopenia have recently been shown to form a spectrum of disorders resulting from mutations in the Wiskott-Aldrich syndrome protein gene at band Xp11-12.[36] The molecular basis for most of the remaining rare inherited causes of neonatal thrombocytopenia, such as thrombocytopenia absent radius syndrome, remains to be identified. A full discussion of these conditions (Table 1) is beyond the scope of this article but they are well covered in a recent review by Geddis.[36]

Aneuploidy

Thrombocytopenia is also recognised in association with various chromosomal abnormalities. Hohlfield et al.[37] found thrombocytopenia present in fetuses with trisomies 18 (86%), 13 (31%) and 21 (6%), as well as triploidy (75%) and Turner syndrome (31%). Usually, the thrombocytopenia is not severe. The mechanism of the thrombocytopenia is not well established though in many cases it is associated with polycythaemia and neutropenia and the mechanism may be similar to the decreased production seen in placental insufficiency (see below).

THROMBOCYTOPENIA SECONDARY TO CHRONIC AND ACUTE HYPOXIA

Placental insufficiency

Neonates with intra-uterine growth restriction have a number of distinctive haematological abnormalities.[19] They are thrombocytopenic and neutropenic and have evidence of increased erythropoiesis (polycythaemia and/or vastly increased numbers of circulating nucleated red cells).[19] The same pattern of abnormalities occurs in a number of conditions: maternal disorders (including pre-eclampsia, hypertension and diabetes mellitus), and fetal disorders manifesting as 'idiopathic' intra-uterine growth restriction. Erythropoietin levels are increased in affected fetuses and neonates and the severity of the haematological abnormalities correlates both with serum erythropoietin levels and with the severity of placental insufficiency.[19]

We and others have shown that megakaryopoiesis is severely impaired at birth in such neonates (as shown by a marked reduction in circulating megakaryocytes and their precursor and progenitor cells) and that this is likely to be the principal reason for the neonatal thrombocytopenia, since there is no evidence of increased platelet destruction/consumption.[14,19] These patients also exhibit significantly raised plasma thrombopoietin levels at the height of their thrombocytopenia, a finding which is increasingly recognised to occur only during hypo-regenerative thrombocytopenias.[7,8] As both the megakaryocyte progenitor abnormalities and the raised thrombopoietin levels resolve in tandem with platelet recovery, these findings suggest that these neonates have underlying impaired platelet production originating in fetal life. The precise haemopoietic mechanism responsible for these abnormalities remains uncertain, although a number of lines of evidence point to disruption of the commitment of fetal multipotent haemopoietic progenitor cells to megakaryopoiesis in association with raised erythropoietin levels.[19]

Asphyxia

Perinatal asphyxia is manifested by the clinical picture of fetal distress, acidaemia, low Apgar scores and encephalopathy. Thrombocytopenia occurs in up to 30% of affected neonates. The thrombocytopenia is both severe and prolonged and is principally secondary to disseminated intramuscular coagulation.[38]

MANAGEMENT OF NEONATAL THROMBOCYTOPENIA

IDENTIFYING THE CAUSE OF THE THROMBOCYTOPENIA

As well as causing significant morbidity, thrombocytopenia can often be the presenting feature of significant disease and, despite its frequency on neonatal units, it is important to try and identify the cause. As mentioned above, thrombocytopenia in the newborn typically takes one of a number of well-defined patterns. Recognition of these patterns helps to identify those neonates in need of urgent investigation and treatment. The causes in term and preterm infants are usually different.

A simple algorithm for the management of thrombocytopenia in preterm neonates is shown in Figure 1. For neonates who develop thrombocytopenia within the first 72 h of life, the majority of mild-to-moderate cases will be associated with placental insufficiency and so there will be a history of

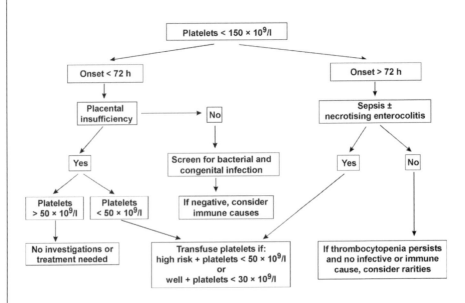

Fig. 1 Management of thrombocytopenia in preterm neonates.

maternal pre-eclampsia, hypertension or diabetes and/or of intra-uterine growth restriction. Unless the thrombocytopenia is severe (platelets < 50 x 10^9/l), or fails to resolve within 10 days, there is usually need for further investigations. However, a platelet count of < 50 x 10^9/l or a persistent thrombocytopenia should prompt further investigation to exclude infection and, if within the first 2 weeks of life, immune causes. Late-onset thrombocytopenia (developing after 72 h of age) in preterm neonates is due to sepsis or necrotising enterocolitis in the vast majority of cases.

The first step in identifying the diagnosis of the cause of thrombocytopenia in a term baby is to consider whether the baby is well or sick. In well, term babies the usual cause is neonatal alloimmune thrombocytopenia (for investigation, see above). In term babies who are unwell, the usual cause is perinatal infection or asphyxia or congenital infection. Aneuploidy may be suspected because of associated anomalies. Where these causes have been excluded and thrombocytopenia persists the baby should be investigated for inherited thrombocytopenias (Table 1). This usually requires bone marrow examination and advice from a paediatric haematologist should be sought.

TREATMENT OF NEONATAL THROMBOCYTOPENIA: THE ROLE OF PLATELET TRANSFUSION

Apart from the specific treatments for immune thrombocytopenias mentioned above, treatment depends upon: (i) treatment of the underlying cause (*e.g.* sepsis); and/or (ii) platelet transfusion. There are no controlled studies for the treatment of significant neonatal thrombocytopenia and only one controlled trial[39] of platelet transfusion to prevent bleeding in neonates with mild or moderate thrombocytopenia (*i.e.* platelet count > 50 x 10^9/l); not surprisingly, this trial failed to show any benefit. Therefore, treatment guidelines and protocols are based on experience, anecdotal evidence and extrapolation from adult studies.[19,23,28]

Platelet transfusions confer one of the highest risks of transfusion-related infections and reactions of all blood products and should be used sparingly.[28] There is a lack of evidence that platelet transfusion improves outcome and what studies there are show no benefit in higher cut-off points for transfusion.[23,28,40] The authors follow the recent British Committee for Standards in Haematology guidelines which recommend a cut-off for platelet transfusion of 30 x 10^9/l in the stable neonate with no bleeding; in the presence of complicating factors, it is recommended to keep the count above 50 x 10^9/.[28] These guidelines take into account the clinical condition of the neonate and the rate of fall of the platelet count as well as the absolute count while recognising that precise definitions of clinical instability are difficult and reflect the predicted risk of bleeding (Table 3). Studies to measure the impact of platelet transfusion more accurately in the management of thrombocytopenic neonates are currently in progress.

HAEMOPOIETIC GROWTH FACTORS

Recombinant human thrombopoietin, the main regulator of megakaryopoiesis in humans, stimulates megakaryocyte precursors from term and preterm neonates

Table 3 Guidelines for platelet transfusion in neonatal thrombocytopenia

Platelet count < 30 x 10^9/l	
In otherwise well infants, including neonatal alloimmune thrombocytopenia, if no bleeding and no family history of intracranial haemorrhage	
Platelet count < 50 x 10^9/l	
In infants with:	Clinical instability
	Concurrent coagulopathy
	Birthweight < 1000 g and age < 1 week
	Previous major bleeding (*e.g.* grade 3/4 intraventricular haemorrhage)
	Current minor bleeding (*e.g.* petechiae)
	Planned surgery or exchange transfusion
	Platelet count falling and likely to fall < 30
	Neonatal alloimmune thrombocytopenia if previous affected sibling with intracranial haemorrhage

Modified from Gibson *et al.*[28]

and it was hoped treatment with recombinant human thrombopoietin might help ameliorate thrombocytopenia in the sick neonate.[5,8] However, the development of neutralising antibodies is common and this, together with the delay of up to a week before a rise in the platelet count is seen, is likely to severely limit its use.[23] Interleukin-11, another cytokine which stimulates megakaryopoiesis and platelet production *in vivo* and *in vitro*, is also available in recombinant form for administration to humans. However, there are no data about recombinant interleukin-11 in neonatal thrombocytopenia and it remains a potential therapeutic prospect for the future.[23]

Key points for clinical practice

- Neonatal thrombocytopenia is one of the commonest haematological abnormalities in the neonatal intensive care unit. Around one-third of preterm neonates cared for in the neonatal intensive care unit develop thrombocytopenia at some point during their stay.

- Although the healthy fetus and neonate can generate and maintain platelet counts at adult levels from early in gestation, differences in fetal and neonatal megakaryopoiesis predispose the sick neonate to thrombocytopenia.

- The normal platelet count in neonates, regardless of gestation, is > 150 x 10^9/l.

- The cause and mechanism of neonatal thrombocytopenia can often be identified by the time at which the thrombocytopenia develops and the associated clinical features.

(continued)

- Early-onset thrombocytopenia in preterm neonates is most commonly due to disorders associated with placental insufficiency, particularly intra-uterine growth restriction, maternal hypertension and diabetes; this is usually mild-moderate, self-limiting and does not require treatment.

- Late-onset thrombocytopenia in preterm neonates is most commonly due sepsis and necrotising enterocolitis; this is often severe (platelets < 50 x 10⁹/l) and requires treatment by platelet transfusion.

- The most common cause of severe thrombocytopenia in a well, term baby is neonatal alloimmune thrombocytopenia. This causes intracranial haemorrhage in up to 20% of neonates and maybe associated with long-term neurodevelopmental problems.

- Congenital infections, particularly due to cytomegalovirus, are an important cause of persistent thrombocytopenia; this may take several months to resolve.

- The genetic basis of many forms of inherited thrombocytopenia has now been identified and key genes in megakaryocyte development are often involved. Examples include mutations of the thrombopoietin receptor (*c-mpl*) and the megakaryocyte transcription factor GATA1.

- There are no evidence-based guidelines for platelet transfusion for neonatal thrombocytopenia and treatment recommendations are based on consensus opinion and experience. Such guidelines are needed in order to assess properly the indications for platelet transfusion, the optimum dose and schedule of administration and the therapeutic effects of platelet transfusion in the short- and long-term.

References

1. Marshall CJ, Thrasher AJ. The embryonic origins of human haematopoiesis. *Br J Haematol* 2001; **112**: 838–850.
2. Hann IM. *Development of Blood in the Fetus*. London: Baillière Tindall, 1991; 1–28.
3. Forestier F, Daffos F, Catherine N, Renard M, Andreux JP. Developmental hematopoiesis in normal human fetal blood. *Blood* 1991; **77**: 2360–2363.
4. Burrows RF, Kelton JG. Fetal thrombocytopenia and its relation to maternal thrombocytopenia. *N Engl J Med* 1993; **329**: 1463–1466.
5. Murray NA, Watts TL, Roberts IAG. Thrombopoietin in the fetus and neonate. *Early Hum Dev* 2000; **59**: 1–12.
6. Challier C, Cocault L, Berthier R *et al*. The cytoplasmic domain of Mpl receptor transduces exclusive signals in embryonic and fetal hematopoietic cells. *Blood* 2002; **100**: 2063–2070.
7. Sola MC, Juul SE, Meng YG *et al*. Thrombopoietin (Tpo) in the fetus and neonate: Tpo concentrations in preterm and term neonates, and organ distribution of Tpo and its receptor (c-mpl) during human fetal development. *Early Hum Dev* 1999; **53**: 239–250.
8. Watts TL, Murray NA, Roberts IAG. Thrombopoietin has a primary role in the regulation of platelet production in preterm babies. *Pediatr Res* 1999; **46**: 28–32.

9. Sola MC, Calhoun DA, Hutson AD, Christensen RD. Plasma thrombopoietin concentrations in thrombocytopenic and non-thrombocytopenic patients in a neonatal intensive care unit. *Br J Haematol* 1999; **104**: 90–92.

10. de Sauvage FJ, Carver-Moore K, Luoh SM *et al.* Physiological regulation of early and late stages of megakaryocytopoiesis by thrombopoietin. *J Exp Med* 1996; **183**: 651–656.

11. Gurbuxani S, Vyas P, Crispino JD. Recent insights into the mechanisms of myeloid leukemogenesis in Down syndrome. *Blood* 2004; **103**: 399–406.

12. de Alarcon PA, Graeve JL. Analysis of megakaryocyte ploidy in fetal bone marrow biopsies using a new adaptation of the feulgen technique to measure DNA content and estimate megakaryocyte ploidy from biopsy specimens. *Pediatr Res* 1996; **39**: 166–170.

13. Paulus JM, Debili N, Larbret F, Levin J, Vainchenker W. Thrombopoietin responsiveness reflects the number of doublings undergone by megakaryocyte progenitors. *Blood* 2004; **104**: 2291–2298.

14. Murray NA, Roberts IAG. Circulating megakaryocytes and their progenitors in early thrombocytopenia in preterm neonates. *Pediatr Res* 1996; **40**: 112–119.

15. Burrows RF, Kelton JG. Incidentally detected thrombocytopenia in healthy mothers and their infants. *N Engl J Med* 1988; **319**: 142–145.

16. Sainio S Jarvenpaa AL, Renlund M, Riikonen S, Teramo K, Kekomaki R. Thrombocytopenia in term infants: a population-based study. *Obstet Gynecol* 2000; **95**: 441–446.

17. de Moerloose P, Boehlen F, Extermann P, Hohfeld P. Neonatal thrombocytopenia: incidence and characterisation of maternal antiplatelet antibodies by MAIPA assay. *Br J Haematol* 1998; **100**: 735–740.

18. Castle V, Andrew M, Kelton J, Giron D, Johnston M, Carter C. Frequency and mechanism of neonatal thrombocytopenia. *J Pediatr* 1986; **108**: 749–755.

19. Murray NA, Howarth LJ, McCloy MP, Letsky EA, Roberts IAG. Platelet transfusion in the management of severe thrombocytopenia in neonatal intensive care unit patients. *Transfus Med* 2002; **12**: 35–41.

20. Kahn DJ, Richardson DK, Billett HH. Inter-NICU variation in rates and management of thrombocytopenia among very low birth-weight infants. *J Perinatol* 2003; **23**: 312–316.

21. Kahn DJ, Richardson DK, Billett HH. Association of thrombocytopenia and delivery method with intraventricular hemorrhage among very-low-birth-weight infants. *Am J Obstet Gynecol* 2002; **186**: 109–116.

22. Jhawar BS, Ranger A, Steven D, Del Maestro RF. Risk factors for intracranial hemorrhage among full-term infants: a case-control study. *Neurosurgery* 2003; **52**: 581–590.

23. Roberts I, Murray NA. Neonatal thrombocytopenia: causes and management. *Arch Dis Child* 2003; **88**: F359–F364.

24. Watts TL, Roberts IAG. Haematological abnormalities in the growth-restricted infant. *Semin Neonatol* 1999; **4**: 41–54.

25. Kaplan C. Alloimmune thrombocytopenia of the fetus and the newborn. *Blood Rev* 2002; **16**: 69–72.

26. Davoren A, Curtis BR, Aster RH, McFarland JG. Human platelet antigen-specific alloantibodies implicated in 1162 cases of neonatal alloimmune thrombocytopenia. *Transfusion* 2004; **44**: 1220–1225.

27. Williamson LM, Hackett G, Rennie J *et al.* The natural history of fetomaternal alloimmunization to the platelet-specific antigen HPA-1a (PlA1, Zwa) as determined by antenatal screening. *Blood* 1998; **92**: 2280–2287.

28. Gibson BE, Todd A, Roberts I *et al.* and British Committee for Standards in Haematology Transfusion Task Force: Writing group. Transfusion guidelines for neonates and older children. *Br J Haematol* 2004; **124**; 433–453.

29. Kelton JG. Idiopathic thrombocytopenic purpura complicating pregnancy. *Blood Rev* 2002; **16**: 43–46.

30. Webert KE, Mittal R, Sigouin C, Heddle NM, Kelton JG. A retrospective 11-year analysis of obstetric patients with idiopathic thrombocytopenic purpura. *Blood* 2003; **102**: 4306–4311.

31. Colarizi P, Fiorucci P, Caradonna A, Ficuccilli F, Mancuso M, Papoff P. Circulating thrombopoietin levels in neonates with infection. *Acta Paediatr* 1999; **88**: 332–337.

32. Murray NA, Watts TL, Roberts IAG. Inhibition of megakaryocytopoiesis in 'late', sepsis-associated thrombocytopenia in preterm babies. *Blood* 1999; **94 (Suppl 1)**: 450a.

33. Miura E, Procianoy RS, Bittar C *et al*. A randomised, double-masked, placebo-controlled trial of recombinant granulocyte colony-stimulating factor administration to preterm infants with the clinical signs of early-onset sepsis. *Pediatrics* 2001; **107**: 30–35.
34. Boppana SB, Fowler KB, Britt WJ, Stagno S, Pass RF. Symptomatic congenital cytomegalovirus infection in infants born to mothers with pre-existing immunity to cytomegalovirus. *Pediatrics* 1999; **104**, 55–60.
35. McAuley J, Boyer KM, Patel D *et al*. Early and longitudinal evaluations of treated infants and children and untreated historical patients with congenital toxoplasmosis: the Chicago Collaborative Treatment Trial. *Clin Infect Dis* 1994; **18**: 38–72.
36. Geddis AE, Kaushansky K. Inherited thrombocytopenias: toward a molecular understanding of disorders of platelet production. *Curr Opin Pediatr* 2004; **16**: 15–22.
37. Hohlfeld P, Forestier F, Kaplan C, Tissot JD, Daffos F. Fetal thrombocytopenia: a retrospective survey of 5194 fetal blood samplings. *Blood* 1994; **84**: 1851–1856.
38. Debillon T, Daoud P, Durand P *et al*. Whole-body cooling after perinatal asphyxia: a pilot study in term neonates. *Dev Med Child Neurol* 2003; **45**: 17–23.
39. Andrew M, Vegh P, Caco C *et al*. A randomized, controlled trial of platelet transfusions in thrombocytopenic premature infants. *J Pediatr* 1993; **123**: 285–291.
40. Del Vecchio A, Sola MC, Theriaque DW *et al*. Platelet transfusions in the neonatal intensive care unit: factors predicting which patients will require multiple transfusions. *Transfusion* 2001; **41**: 803–808.

Jon F. Watchko M. Jeffrey Maisels

9

Management of jaundice in preterm infants

Hyperbilirubinaemia in preterm infants is more prevalent, its severity more pronounced, and its course more protracted than in term neonates,[1] as a result of exaggerated neonatal red cell, hepatic and gastrointestinal immaturity. The postnatal maturation of hepatic bilirubin uptake and conjugation may also be slower in premature infants.[2] In addition, a delay in the initiation of enteral feedings so common in the clinical management of sick premature newborns may limit intestinal flow and bacterial colonisation resulting in a further enhancement of bilirubin enterohepatic circulation.[2] These developmental and clinical phenomena contribute to the greater degree (maximum serum bilirubin) and duration (age at peak bilirubin) of neonatal jaundice in premature infants (Fig. 1).

Despite the near universal finding of clinical jaundice in the preterm infant, kernicterus has virtually disappeared in post mortem series of premature neonates,[3] and post-kernicteric bilirubin encephalopathy and central neural hearing loss related to neonatal hyperbilirubinaemia have not emerged as important clinical sequelae in neurodevelopmental follow-up of premature infants.[2] Yet kernicterus has occurred in preterm infants at low bilirubin levels and in the absence of acute neurological signs.[4,5] Investigators have suggested that moderate hyperbilirubinaemia (total serum bilirubin [TSB] levels higher than 10–14 mg/dl [170–239 µmol/l]) may be associated with milder forms of central nervous system dysfunction and sequelae.[6,7] Moreover, two recent

Jon F. Watchko MD (for correspondence)
Division of Neonatology and Developmental Biology, Department of Pediatrics, University of Pittsburgh School of Medicine, Magee-Women's Hospital, 300 Halket Street, Pittsburgh, PA 15213, USA
E-mail: jwatchko@mail.magee.edu

M. Jeffrey Maisels MB BCh
Department of Pediatrics, William Beaumont Hospital, Royal Oak, MI 48073, USA

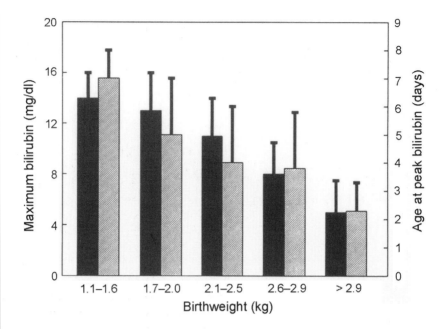

Fig. 1 Bar graph demonstrating maximum bilirubin levels (black bars, mg/dl) and age at peak bilirubin level (grey bars, days) in premature infants as a function of birth weight (kg). These data reflect the natural history of postnatal hyperbilirubinaemia in the absence of any therapeutic intervention (*i.e.* phototherapy or exchange transfusion). Adapted from *BMJ* 1954; **2**: 1263–1265.

reports of kernicterus in preterm neonates in whom bilirubin levels ranged from 8.7 to 14.7 (148–251 μmol/l) have raised renewed concerns about low-bilirubin kernicterus in the premature infant.[5,8]

The literature on bilirubin-induced neurological injury in the jaundiced preterm neonate reveals a complexity that is far greater than suggested by a simple *a priori* cause and effect relation between TSB and neuronal damage,[9] leaving neonatologists in a clinical quandary with respect to the management of neonatal hyperbilirubinaemia in the premature infant.[10] There is, nevertheless, little doubt that kernicterus is currently a very rare event in premature infants hospitalised in neonatal intensive care units.[3] This may be the result of overall improvements in care and/or of the fairly aggressive use of phototherapy. Randomised clinical studies such as that being carried out currently by the National Institute of Child Health and Human Development Neonatal Research Network designed to compare aggressive with conservative use of phototherapy and exchange transfusion in extremely low birth weight infants will help to define more clearly the risks of hyper-bilirubinaemia in premature neonates and the indications for clinical interventions.[11]

JAUNDICE MANAGEMENT GUIDELINES IN PRETERM NEONATES

The inability to relate specific TSB levels in premature infants to developmental outcome or pathological kernicterus has made the framing of guidelines for the

Table 1 Guidelines for the use of phototherapy and exchange transfusion in low birth weight infants based on birth weight[a]

Birth weight (g)	Total bilirubin level (mg/dl [μmol/l])[b]	
	Phototherapy[c]	Exchange transfusion[d]
≤ 1500	5–8 (85–140)	13–16 (220–275)
1500–1999	8–12 (140–200)	16–18 (275–300)
2000–2499	11–14 (190–240)	18–20 (300–340)

[a]Note that these guidelines reflect ranges used in neonatal intensive care units. They cannot take into account all possible situations. Lower bilirubin levels should be used for infants who are sick (*e.g.* presence of sepsis, acidosis, hypoalbuminaemia) or have haemolytic disease.

[b]Consider initiating therapy at these levels. Range allows discretion based on clinical conditions or other circumstances. Note that bilirubin levels refer to total serum bilirubin concentrations. Direct reacting or conjugated bilirubin levels should not be subtracted from the total.

[c]Used at these levels and in therapeutic doses, phototherapy should, with few exceptions, eliminate the need for exchange transfusions.

[d]Levels for exchange transfusion assume that bilirubin continues to rise or remains at these levels despite intensive phototherapy.

From Maisels.[12]

Table 2 Guidelines for use of phototherapy and exchange transfusion in preterm infants based on gestational age

	Total bilirubin level (mg/dl [μmol/l]) Exchange transfusion		
Gestational age	Phototherapy	Sick*	Well
36	14.6 (250)	17.5 (300)	20.5 (350)
32	8.8 (150)	14.6 (250)	17.5 (300)
28	5.8 (100)	11.7 (200)	14.6 (250)
24	4.7 (80)	8.8 (150)	11.7 (200)

*Rhesus disease, perinatal asphyxia, hypoxia, acidosis, hypercapnia; from Ives.[13]

Table 3 Guidelines for exchange transfusion in low birth weight infants based on total bilirubin (mg/dl) and bilirubin/albumin ratio (mg/g)

	Birth weight (g)			
	< 1250	1250–1499	1500–1999	2000–2499
Standard risk	13	15	17	18
Or bilirubin/albumin ratio	5.2	6.0	6.8	7.2
High risk[a]	10	13	15	17
Or bilirubin/albumin ratio	4.0	5.2	6.0	6.8

*Exchange transfusion at whichever comes first.

[a]Risk factors: Apgar < 3 at 5 min; PaO_2 < 40 mmHg > 2 h, pH < 7.15 > 1 h; birth weight < 1000 g, haemolysis; clinical or central nervous system deterioration; total protein < 4 g/dl or albumin < 2.5 g/dl. *From Ahlfors.*[14]

use of phototherapy and exchange transfusion in these infants a capricious exercise at best and one for which no claim of an 'evidence-base' can be made. Reference to Tables 1–3 illustrates a range of TSB levels for intervention in varying circumstances.[12–14] These guidelines are provided by different experts none of whom, we believe, would make any claim for the greater validity of one approach versus another. The aim of treatment is to prevent bilirubin-related neurodevelopmental handicap while not causing harm. The almost complete disappearance of pathological kernicterus in this population suggests that if this is the result of fairly aggressive phototherapy, used on a sliding scale as shown in Tables 1–3, we must be doing something right. On the other hand, both the absence of any other evidence (in the form of controlled clinical trials) to support this approach[2,11] and the possibility that phototherapy might have other, less desirable consequences, should give us pause.

Bilirubin is a powerful antioxidant and may have a physiological role as an antioxidant in the human neonate.[15] It has also been suggested that keeping TSB levels low with phototherapy (and thus reducing the antioxidant level) could facilitate the development of retinopathy of prematurity. In a study of 157 23–26-week gestation infants, however, no relationship was found between TSB levels and retinopathy of prematurity.[16] More than 90% of extremely low birth weight infants (birth weights < 1000 g) receive phototherapy, and concern for the possible negative consequences of aggressive phototherapy has led the National Institute of Child Health and Human Development Neonatal Research Network to initiate a prospective randomised trial to compare aggressive with conservative phototherapy in these infants.[11] The TSB levels for intervention with phototherapy and exchange transfusion in this on-going trial are shown in Table 4. The primary outcome will be death or neurodevelopmental impairment at 18–22 months corrected age. The results of this study should provide important information about the risks and benefits of phototherapy in this vulnerable population.

Tables 1–3 provide suggested guidelines for the management of hyper-bilirubinaemia in low birth weight infants. Phototherapy is generally used according to a sliding scale – the lower the birth weight or gestation, the lower the TSB level at which phototherapy is instituted although there is little good evidence to support this practice except, perhaps, for the influence of gestation on bilirubin-albumin

Table 4 Guidelines for initiating phototherapy and exchange transfusions – NICHD Neonatal Research Network Trial

Birth weight	Aggressive management		Conservative management	
	Phototx begins	Exchange transfusion	Phototx begins	Exchange transfusion
501–750 g	ASAP after enrolment	≥ 13.0 mg/dl	≥ 8.0 mg/dl	≥ 13.0 mg/dl
751–1000 g	ASAP after enrolment	≥ 15.0 mg/dl	≥ 10.0 mg/dl	≥ 15.0 mg/dl

Enrolment is expected within the period 12–36 h after birth, preferably between 12 and 24 h. From Morris.[11]

binding.[17] These guidelines reflect ranges used in different neonatal intensive care units and cannot take into account all possible situations.

CLINICAL USE OF THE BILIRUBIN/ALBUMIN RATIO

Bilirubin is transported in the plasma tightly bound to albumin and the portion that is unbound or loosely bound can more readily leave the intravascular space and cross the intact blood–brain barrier. Elevations of unbound bilirubin have been associated with kernicterus in sick, preterm newborns.[18] In addition, elevated unbound bilirubin concentrations are more closely associated than TSB levels with transient abnormalities in the audiometric brain stem response in preterm infants.[19] There are, however, no contemporary long-term studies relating unbound bilirubin concentrations in low birth-weight infants to developmental outcome. In one follow-up of 224 infants born in 1974–1976 with birth weights below 2000 g and evaluated at age 6 years, no relation was found between measures of bilirubin–albumin binding and IQ scores.[20] In addition, clinical laboratory measurement of unbound bilirubin is not generally available.

The ratio of bilirubin (mg/dl) to albumin (g/dl) does correlate with measured unbound bilirubin in newborns[14] and has been used as an approximate surrogate for the measurement of unbound bilirubin.[14] It must be recognised, however, that albumin binding capacity varies significantly between newborns,[14,21] is impaired in sick infants,[21] and increases with increasing gestational age[17] and post-natal age.[17] Furthermore, the risk of bilirubin encephalopathy is not simply a function of the TSB level or the concentration of unbound bilirubin but is a combination of both, *i.e.* the total amount of bilirubin available (the miscible pool of bilirubin) as well as the tendency of bilirubin to enter the tissue (the unbound bilirubin concentration).[14] An additional factor is the susceptibility of the cells of the central nervous system to damage by bilirubin.[22] The bilirubin/albumin ratio can, therefore, be used together with, but not in lieu of, the TSB level as an additional factor in determining the need for exchange transfusion (Table 3).[14]

EXCHANGE TRANSFUSION

Exchange transfusion was the first intervention to permit effective control of hyperbilirubinaemia and thus, prevent kernicterus during the severe jaundice associated with the immune-mediated haemolysis of Rh isoimmunisation. Often such infants were preterm. In addition to the immediate control of hyperbilirubinaemia, an exchange transfusion in immune-mediated haemolytic disease also achieves: (i) the removal of antibody-coated red blood cells (a source of 'potential' bilirubin); (ii) the correction of anaemia (if present); and (iii) the removal of maternal antibody.[23] Exchange transfusions are most readily performed via the umbilical vein using an umbilical catheter inserted just far enough to obtain free flow of blood (usually no more than the distance between the xiphoid process and umbilicus). The 'push-pull' method with a single syringe and special four-way stopcock assembly permits a single operator to complete the procedure.[23] Fresh citrate-phosphate-dextrose blood (< 72-h old and devoid of the offending antigen in the case of immune-mediated haemolytic disease) cross-matched to the infant should be used. Although the risk for graft-versus-host disease following an exchange transfusion is extremely rare, blood for exchange transfusion should be irradiated. The blood should be warmed to body temperature by a blood/fluid warmer. The actual exchange should be performed slowly in aliquots of 5–10 cc/kg body weight with each withdrawal-infusion cycle approximating 3-min duration.[23] During the exchange, the infants vital signs should be monitored closely, including ECG, respiration, oxygen saturation, temperature, and blood pressure. Post exchange studies should include: bilirubin, haemoglobin, platelet count, ionised calcium, serum electrolytes, and serum glucose.

COMPLICATIONS OF EXCHANGE TRANSFUSION

Sick, preterm infants are much more likely than term infants to experience a serious complication of exchange transfusion, such as an arrhythmia, thrombosis, thrombocytopenia, nercotising enterocolitis and infection among others,[23] or to die during or soon after the procedure.[24] In a US study[25] of 331 exchange transfusions there was 1 death (a rate of 0.3/100 procedures; 95% confidence limits [CL] 0, 0.9) and significant morbidity in 5%. In 1472 exchange transfusions, Hove and Siimes identified 4 deaths 'possibly related' to the procedure,[26] a rate of 0.3/100 procedures (95% CL; 0, 0.5). Jackson[24] reviewed the records of the Children's Hospital Medical Center and the University of

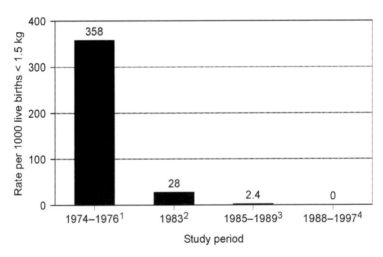

Fig. 2 Number of infants in different populations with birth weight < 1500 g who received exchange transfusions between 1974 and 1997. Note 1. A total of 215 newborns < 1500 g in the NICHD Cooperative Phototherapy Trial assigned to the control group (did not receive phototherapy). Seventy-seven of 215 patients (35.8%) received a total of 161 exchange transfusions. In the phototherapy group, 17 of 196 (8.7%) infants received exchange transfusions. These data are included to illustrate the frequency of exchange transfusion before the introduction of phototherapy.[31] Note 2. Of a total of 1338 live births < 1500 g in The Netherlands (1983), 37 infants (2.8%) required at least one exchange transfusion (from van de Boor et al.[6]). Note 3. Of 833 live births (500–1500 g) in a 17-county region in North Carolina, two infants required an exchange transfusion (0.24%) (from O'Shea et al.[31]). Note 4. No exchange transfusions were performed in 1213 live births < 1500 g at William Beaumont Hospital, Royal Oak, MI between 1988 and 1997 (*from Maisels*[28]).[Reprinted by permission from *Journal of Perinatology* 2001; **21**: S93–S97, Macmillan Publishers Ltd.]

Washington Medical Center in Seattle, Washington, for the 15-year period 1980–1995, during which 106 infants had an exchange transfusion. Of these, 81 were healthy and there were no deaths in these infants although one child developed severe NEC requiring surgery. There were 25 sick newborns; 3 had serious complications from the exchange transfusion and 2 (8%) of these infants died (95% CL; 0, 19%). In three additional infants, deaths were considered 'possibly due' to the exchange transfusion so that the mortality rate could have been as high as 20%. Four surviving infants had permanent serious sequelae – 1 of the 80 surviving well infants and 3 of 20 (15%) sick infants (95% CL; 0, 31%). A more recent report also suggests that adverse events are more frequent in exchange transfusions done on preterm infants ≤ 32 weeks' gestation and in infants who have other pre-existing serious neonatal morbidities.[27]

These rates, however, may not be generalisable to the current era. Experience with exchange transfusion is decreasing (Fig. 2)[28] and it is reasonable to assume that, like most procedures, frequency of performance is an important determinant of risk. It is certainly very difficult, if not impossible, to teach paediatric residents in the US to do exchange transfusions and there is legitimate concern regarding our ability to train even neonatal fellows to perform this once-common procedure. Indeed, with newer phototherapy technologies emerging as well as the potential for pharmacological inhibition of bilirubin production[29] exchange transfusion in the neonatal intensive care unit is in danger of becoming extinct. As discussed previously,[9,10] the validity of traditional criteria for exchange transfusion in the low birth weight population has been questioned and the introduction of more effective phototherapy for these infants has rendered much of the debate regarding exchange transfusion in this population moot.[28]

EXCHANGE TRANSFUSION IN PRETERM INFANTS – IMPACT OF PHOTOTHERAPY

Phototherapy, introduced in 1958 by Cremer and colleagues,[30] has had a profound impact in controlling the level of serum bilirubin in preterm neonates markedly reducing the need for exchange transfusions (Fig. 2)[28,31] in the neonatal intensive care unit population of infants weighing < 1500 g. In a cohort of 833 infants with birth weights of 500–1500 g born in North Carolina between 1985 and 1989, only two infants (0.24%) underwent exchange transfusion[31] and at William Beaumont Hospital in Royal Oak, Michigan, between 1988 and 1997 no exchange transfusions were performed in 1213 live births of infants weighing < 1500 g (Fig. 2).[28] Certainly, phototherapy, if used appropriately,[32] is capable of controlling the bilirubin levels in almost all premature infants, with the possible exception of the occasional infant with severe erythroblastosis fetalis or marked bruising. Furthermore, exchange transfusion, when performed at the low bilirubin levels used for treatment in low birth weight infants is very inefficient and is less effective than phototherapy in achieving prolonged reduction of TSB in infants with non-haemolytic jaundice.[33]

PHOTOTHERAPY IN THE PRETERM INFANT

Phototherapy detoxifies bilirubin by converting bilirubin to photo-isomers that are more polar, less lipophilic and readily excreted from the liver into bile

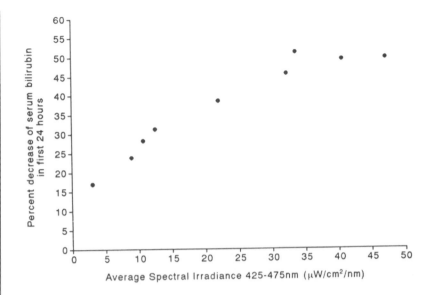

Fig. 3 Relationship between average spectral irradiance and decrease in serum bilirubin concentration. Full-term infants with non-haemolytic hyperbilirubinaemia were exposed to special blue lights (Phillips TL 52/20W) of different intensities. Spectral irradiance was measured as the average of readings at the head, trunk, and knees. Drawn from the data of Tan.[35]

without undergoing conjugation.[34] The photo-isomerisation of bilirubin is fast and likely takes place in blood vessels and/or in the interstitial space.[34] Photodegredation or photo-oxidation of bilirubin to biliverdin plays a minor role in the effectiveness of phototherapy.[34]

USING PHOTOTHERAPY EFFECTIVELY IN THE PREMATURE NEONATE

The effectiveness of phototherapy is determined by several factors including, among others, the: (i) spectrum of light emitted (best wavelengths appear to be in the blue–green region ~425–500 nm); (ii) irradiance of light source (greater the closer the infant is to the light source); and (iii) surface area of infant exposed to the light.[34] As with any therapeutic agent, phototherapy should be administered in an adequate dose and the dose can be measured quite easily using a radiometer obtained from the manufacturer of the phototherapy device. Figure 3 illustrates the dose–response relationship between the irradiance used and the rate at which the TSB level declines in term infants under phototherapy.[35]

Most commonly used phototherapy units deliver enough output in the blue–green region of the visible spectrum to be effective for conventional phototherapy in low birth weight infants.[36] On the other hand, if bilirubin levels approach a range at which exchange transfusion is indicated, then more intensive therapeutic forms of phototherapy should be used.[28] This is achieved by increasing the irradiance and the surface area exposed (see below). The most effective light source currently commercially available is that provided

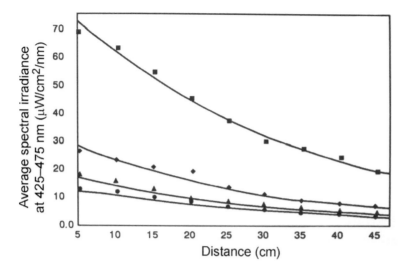

Fig. 4 Effect of light source and distance from the light source to the infant on average spectral irradiance. Measurements were made across the 425–475-nm band using a commercial radiometer (Olympic Bilimeter Mark II). The phototherapy unit was fitted with eight 24-inch fluorescent tubes. Filled squares, indicate special blue, General Electric 20-W F20T12/BB tube; filled diamonds, blue, General Electric 20-W F20T12/B tube; filled triangles, daylight blue, four General Electric 20-W F20T12/B blue tubes and four Sylvania 20-W F20T12/D daylight tubes; and filled circles, daylight, Sylvania 20-W F20T12/D daylight tube. Curves were plotted using linear curve fitting (True Epistat, Epistat Services, Richardson, TX, USA). The best fit is described by the equation $y = Ae^{Bx}$.[32]

by special blue fluorescent tubes.[36] These tubes are labelled F20 T12/BB or PL52/20W and they provide much greater irradiance than regular blue tubes (labelled F20T12/B; Fig. 4). Special blue tubes are more effective because they provide light with wavelengths predominately in the blue–green spectrum, where light penetrates the skin well and is absorbed maximally by bilirubin.[36]

Fibre-optic phototherapy systems have several advantages over conventional phototherapy. Non-distressed neonates can be swaddled or dressed with the fibre-optic blanket placed inside the blankets or clothes. These infants do not need to have their eyes covered (a major benefit to the family), but if the infant is lying (undressed) on a fibre-optic pad, eye patching is advisable. In some studies of low birth weight infants, fibre-optic phototherapy has been as effective as conventional phototherapy[37] but it is less effective when compared with special blue phototherapy lamps.[38]

Spectral irradiance increases dramatically as the distance between the light source and infant decreases and this effect is most significant when special blue tubes are used (Fig. 4). If bilirubin levels are rising in spite of conventional phototherapy (*e.g.* severely bruised infants or those with haemolytic disease), a free-standing bank of special blue fluorescent tubes should be placed about 10 cm from the infant. This proximity is accomplished by placing the fluorescent bank of lights between the radiant warmer and the infant and cannot be achieved when the infant is in an incubator. If halogen spot phototherapy lamps are used, they must not be positioned closer to the infant than recommended by the manufacturer because of the risk of a burn. In addition, if two or more halogen lamps are used they should never be focused on the same area of the infant's skin as this might also cause a burn.

The efficacy of phototherapy is closely related to the surface area of the infant exposed to the phototherapy lights and the simplest way of increasing the surface area exposed is to place fibre-optic pads below the infant with phototherapy lamps above. In preterm infants, this type of 'double phototherapy' is approximately twice as effective as single phototherapy.[38] If this intervention does not produce the desired decrease in the serum bilirubin level, additional exposure can be achieved by lining the sides of the radiant warmer or the incubator with a reflecting material such as white linen or aluminium foil.

Clinical studies comparing intermittent versus continuous phototherapy have produced conflicting results but in most circumstances phototherapy does not need to be continuous. As long as the serum bilirubin level is being controlled, phototherapy can certainly be interrupted during feeding or parental visits. There are conflicting data regarding whether phototherapy significantly increases insensible water loss in preterm infants.[39–41] As we have simple and effective ways of monitoring newborn hydration (such as a daily weight and measurements of electrolytes), there is no indication for routinely providing additional fluids to infants who are receiving phototherapy. They should, of course, be kept adequately hydrated, in part because adequate urine output is important for effective phototherapy. The bilirubin isomer, lumirubin, is excreted in the bile and the urine, and lumirubin excretion appears to be an important element in the bilirubin-lowering function of phototherapy.[36]

COMPLICATIONS OF PHOTOTHERAPY

Significant complications associated with phototherapy are exceptionally rare. Perhaps the most important clinical complication encountered during the use of phototherapy in the low birth weight infant is that associated with the presence of direct hyperbilirubinaemia or cholestatic jaundice (usually following prolonged parental nutrition). When infants with direct hyperbilirubinaemia are exposed to phototherapy, they may develop a dark, greyish-brown discoloration of the skin, serum and urine (the 'bronze baby syndrome'). The pathogenesis of this syndrome is unknown but it is possibly related to the accumulation of porphyrins or other pigments in the plasma in the presence of cholestasis.[42] Although few deleterious consequences of the bronze baby syndrome have been described, two infants with this syndrome who died were shown to have kernicterus at autopsy.[42,43] With the exception of these case reports, there are no other reports of significant complications in infants who develop the bronze baby syndrome although impaired binding of bilirubin to albumin has been detected in three infants with this syndrome[44] and in infants with cholestasis. If there is a need for phototherapy, the presence of direct hyperbilirubinaemia should not be considered a contra-indication to its use, particularly in the sick newborn and, as a rule, the direct serum bilirubin level should not be subtracted from the total bilirubin concentration when decisions are made about initiating phototherapy or an exchange transfusion (Tables 1–3). In infants who develop the bronze baby syndrome, exchange transfusion should be considered if phototherapy does not lower the total serum bilirubin. Because of the paucity of data, however, firm recommendations cannot be made. Rarely, purpuric bullous eruptions have also been described in infants with severe cholestatic jaundice receiving phototherapy.

INTRAVENOUS IMMUNE GLOBULIN

Several studies have demonstrated the effectiveness of early high dose (500–1000 mg/kg) intravenous immune globulin therapy in attenuating haemolysis and resultant hyperbilirubinaemia associated with Coombs positive haemolytic disease (Rh isoimmunisation and ABO in compatibility).[45–47] Indeed, intravenous immune globulin therapy significantly decreased blood carboxyhaemoglobin levels by 24 h post-intravenous immune globulin therapy, a sensitive marker of neonatal haemolysis[46] and a recent systematic review reported that the 'number needed to treat' with intravenous immune globulin therapy in order to prevent one exchange transfusion was low at 2.7 attesting to the efficacy of this intervention.[47] Intravenous immune globulin therapy should be given slowly (over at least 2 h) and can be repeated at 12-h intervals until the bilirubin stabilises.[45]

Key points for clinical practice

- Hyperbilirubinaemia in preterm infants is more prevalent, more severe, and its course more protracted than in term neonates tending to peak at day 5–7.

- Guidelines for the use of phototherapy and exchange transfusion in preterm infants are empirical for which no claim of an 'evidence-base' can be made.

- Phototherapy if used appropriately is capable of controlling bilirubin levels in almost all premature infants with the exception of the occasional infant with severe erythroblastosis fetalis or marked bruising.

- Serious complications of exchange transfusion are more likely in sick, preterm infants than in their healthy term counterparts.

- During an exchange transfusion, the infant's vital signs should be monitored closely, including ECG, respiration, oxygen saturation, temperature, and blood pressure. Post exchange studies should include: bilirubin, haemoglobin, platelet count, ionised calcium, serum electrolytes, and serum glucose.

- The effectiveness of phototherapy is determined by several factors including the: (i) spectrum of light emitted (best wavelengths appear to be in the blue-green region ~425–500 nm); (ii) irradiance of light source (greater the closer the infant is

(continued on next page)

---

to the light source); and (iii) surface area of infant exposed to the light.

- The most effective light source currently commercially available is that provided by special blue fluorescent tube. These tubes are labelled F20 T12/BB or PL52/20W and they provide much greater irradiance than regular blue tubes (labelled F20T12/B).

- Preterm infants on phototherapy should be kept adequately hydrated, in part because adequate urine output is important for effective lumirubin excretion.

- The direct serum bilirubin level should not be subtracted from the total serum bilirubin when decisions are made about initiating phototherapy or an exchange transfusion (Tables 1–3).

- Early high dose (500–1000 mg/kg) intravenous immune globulin is effective in attenuating haemolysis and resultant hyperbilirubinaemia associated with Coombs positive haemolytic disease (Rh isoimmunisation and ABO in compatibility).

- When administered, intravenous immune globulin should be given slowly (over at least 2 h).

References

1. Billing BH, Cole PG, Lathe GH. Increased plasma bilirubin in newborn infants in relation to birth weight. *BMJ* 1954; **2**: 1263–1265.
2. Cashore WJ. Bilirubin and jaundice in the micropremie. *Clin Perinatol* 2000; **27**: 171–179.
3. Watchko J, Claasen D. Kernicterus in premature infants: current prevalence and relationship to NICHD phototherapy study exchange criteria. *Pediatrics* 1994; **93**: 996–999.
4. Gartner LM, Snyder RN, Chabon RS, Bernstein J. Kernicterus: high incidence in premature infants with low serum bilirubin concentrations. *Pediatrics* 1970; **45**: 906–917.
5. Sugama S, Soeda A, Eto Y. Magnetic resonance imaging in three children with kernicterus. *Pediatr Neurol* 2001; **25**: 328–331.
6. van de Bor M, van Zeben-van der Aa TM, Verloove-Vanhorick SP *et al.* Hyperbilirubinemia in very preterm infants and neurodevelopmental outcome at two years of age: results of a national collaborative survey. *Pediatrics* 1989; **83**: 915–920.
7. Scheidt PC, Mellitis ED, Hardy JB, Drage JS, Boggs TR. Toxicity to bilirubin in neonates: infant development during first year in relation to maximum neonatal serum bilirubin concentration. *J Pediatr* 1977; **91**: 292–297.
8. Govaert P, Lequin M, Swarte R *et al.* Changes in globus pallidus with (pre) term kernicterus. *Pediatrics* 2003; **112**: 1256–1263.
9. Ahdab-Barmada M. Neuropathology of kernicterus: definitions and debate. In: Maisels MJ, Watchko JF. (eds) *Neonatal Jaundice*. Amsterdam: Harwood, 2000; 75–88.
10. Watchko JF. The clinical sequelae of hyperbilirubinemia. In: Maisels MJ, Watchko JF. (eds) *Neonatal Jaundice*, Amsterdam: Harwood, 2000; 115–135.
11. Morris B. A randomized trial of aggressive or conservative phototherapy for extremely low birth weight infants. National Institute of Child Health and Development Neonatal Research Network. Personal communication, 2002.
12. Maisels MJ. Jaundice. In: Avery GB, Fletcher MA, MacDonald MG. (eds) *Neonatology: Pathophysiology and Management of the Newborn*. Philadelphia, PA: J.B. Lippincott, 1999; 765–819.
13. Ives NK. Neonatal jaundice. In: Rennie JM, Roberton NRC. (eds) *Textbook of Neonatology*. New York: Churchill Livingstone, 1999; 715–732.

14. Ahlfors CE. Criteria for exchange transfusion in jaundiced newborns. *Pediatrics* 1994; **93**: 488–494.

15. Hegyi T, Goldie E, Hiatt M. The protective role of bilirubin in oxygen radical disease of the preterm infant. *J Perinatol* 1994; **14**: 296–300.

16. DeJonge MH, Khuntia A, Maisels MJ, Bandagi A. Bilirubin levels and severe retinopathy of prematurity in 23–26 week estimated gestational age infants. *J Pediatr* 1999; **135**: 102–104.

17. Ebbesen F, Nyboe J. Postnatal changes in the ability of plasma albumin to bind bilirubin. *Acta Paediatr Scand* 1983; **72**: 665–670.

18. Cashore WJ, Oh W. Unbound bilirubin and kernicterus in low birthweight infants. *Pediatrics* 1982; **69**: 481–485.

19. Amin SB, Ahlfors CE, Orlando MS, Dalzell LE, Merle KS, Guillet R. Bilirubin and serial auditory brainstem responses in premature infants. *Pediatrics* 2001; **107**: 664–670.

20. Scheidt PC, Graubard BI, Nelson KB *et al.* Intelligence at six years in relation to neonatal bilirubin level: follow-up of the National Institute of Child Health and Human Development Clinical Trial of Phototherapy. *Pediatrics* 1991; **87**: 797–805.

21. Cashore WJ. Free bilirubin concentrations and bilirubin-binding affinity in term and preterm infants. *J Pediatr* 1980; **96**: 521–527.

22. Wennberg RP. Cellular basis of bilirubin toxicity. *NY State J Med* 1991; **91**: 493–496.

23. Watchko JF. Exchange transfusion. In: Maisels MJ, Watchko JF. (eds) *Neonatal Jaundice*. Amsterdam: Harwood, 2000; 169–176.

24. Jackson JC. Adverse events associated with exchange transfusion in healthy and ill newborns. *Pediatrics* 1997; 99: 5 URL: <http//www.pediatrics.org/cgi/content/full/99/5/e7>.

25. Keenan WJ, Novak KK, Sutherland JM *et al.* Morbidity and mortality associated with exchange transfusion. *Pediatrics (Suppl)* 1985; **75**: 417–421.

26. Hovi L, Siimes MA. Exchange transfusion with fresh heparinized blood is a safe procedure: experiences from 1069 newborns. *Acta Paediatr Scand* 1985; **74**: 360–365.

27. Petra K, Storfer-Isser A, Siner B, Moore J, Hack M. Adverse events associated with neonatal exchange transfusion in the 1990s. *J Pediatr* 2004; **144**: 626–631.

28. Maisels MJ. Phototherapy – traditional and nontraditional. *J Perinatol* 2001; **21**: S93–S97.

29. Kappas A, Drummond G, Henschke C *et al.* Direct comparison of Sn-mesoporphyrin, an inhibitor of bilirubin production, and phototherapy in controlling hyperbilirubinemia in term and near-term newborns. *Pediatrics* 1995; **95**: 468–474.

30. Cremer RJ, Perryman PW, Richards DH. Influence of light on the hyperbilirubinemia of infants. *Lancet* 1958; **1**: 1094–1097.

31. O'Shea TM, Dillard RG, Klinepeter KD *et al.* Serum bilirubin levels, intracranial hemorrhage, and the risk of developmental problems in very low birth weight infants. *Pediatrics* 1992; **90**: 888–892.

32. Maisels MJ. Why use homeopathic doses of phototherapy? *Pediatrics* 1996; **98**: 283–287.

33. Tan KL. Comparison of the effectiveness of phototherapy and exchange transfusion in the management of nonhemolytic neonatal hyperbilirubinemia. *J Pediatr* 1975; **87**: 609–612.

34. Maisels MJ. Phototherapy. In: Maisels MJ, Watchko JF. (eds) *Neonatal Jaundice*. London: Harwood, 2000; 177–204.

35. Tan KL. The pattern of bilirubin response to phototherapy for neonatal hyperbilirubinemia. *Pediatr Res* 1982; **16**: 670–674.

36. Ennever JF. Blue light, green light, white light, more light: treatment of neonatal jaundice. *Clin Perinatol* 1990; **17**: 467–481.

37. Costello SA, Nyikal J, Yu VY, McCloud P. BiliBlanket phototherapy system versus conventional phototherapy: a randomized controlled trial in preterm infants [see comments]. *J Paediatr Child Health* 1995; **31**: 11–13.

38. Donzelli GP, Moroni M, Pratesi S, Rapisardi G, Agati G, Fusi F. Fibreoptic phototherapy in the management of jaundice in low birthweight neonates. *Acta Paediatr* 1996; **85**: 366–370.

39. Kjartansson S, Hammarlund K, Sedin G. Insensible water loss from the skin during phototherapy in term and preterm infants. *Acta Paediatr* 1992; **81**: 764–768.

40. Maayan-Metzger A, Yosipovitch G, Hadad E, Sirota L. Transepidermal water loss and

skin hydration in preterm infants during phototherapy. *Am J Perinatol* 2001; **18**: 393–396.

41. Grunhagen DJ, De Boer MGJ, De Beaufort AJ, Walter FJ. Transepidermal water loss during halogen spotlight phototherapy in preterm infants. *Pediatr Res* 2002; **51**: 402–405.

42. Rubaltelli FF, Da Riol R, D'Amore E, Jori G. The bronze baby syndrome: evidence of increased tissue concentration of copper porphyrins. *Acta Paediatr* 1996; **85**: 381–384.

43. Clark CF, Torii S, Hamamoto Y, Kaito H. The 'bronze baby' syndrome: postmortem data. *J Pediatr* 1976; **88**: 461–464.

44. Ebbesen F. Low reserve albumin for binding of bilirubin in neonates with deficiency of bilirubin excretion and bronze baby syndrome. *Acta Paediatr Scand* 1982; **71**: 415–410.

45. Hammerman C, Kaplan M. Recent developments in the management of neonatal hyperbilirubinemia. *NeoReviews* 2000; **1**: e19–e24.

46. Hammerman C, Vreman HJ, Kaplan M, Stevenson DK. Intravenous immune globulin in neonatal immune hemolytic disease: does it reduce hemolysis. *Acta Paediatr* 1996; **85**: 1351–1353.

47. Gottstein R, Cooke RWI. Systematic review of intravenous immunoglobulin in haemolytic disease of the newborn. *Arch Dis Child* 2003; **88**: F6–F10.

Mirna Chehade Scott H. Sicherer

10

Infantile food protein-induced enterocolitis syndrome

Food protein-induced enterocolitis syndrome is a type of adverse immune response to food (food allergy) that occurs primarily in infants and is most commonly caused by cow's milk protein. The primary symptoms are essentially non-specific, and include vomiting, diarrhoea, and failure to thrive. This symptom complex potentially overlaps a wide variety of disorders with a multitude of aetiologies such as infection and metabolic disorders. Interestingly, the most common misdiagnosis a paediatrician will make for a child eventually diagnosed with this syndrome is bacterial sepsis. This mis-identification of a food-allergic reaction is understandable because when the causal food is re-introduced to a child with food protein-induced enterocolitis syndrome after symptoms improve, there is a characteristic delayed onset of a symptom complex of severe and repetitive vomiting, lethargy, elevated white blood cell count, sometimes acidemia and cyanosis caused by methaemoglobinaemia, with eventual onset of diarrhoea; these symptoms pose a clinical presentation that fully overlaps the presentation of bacterial sepsis. To make the diagnosis even more elusive, the astute clinician who considers a possible food-allergic reaction and tests the infant for allergic responses with typical methods such as a serum test for IgE antibody to milk or other suspected triggers, will discover negative results even though the reaction is, indeed, food-related. Second episodes are, therefore, a common problem prior to confirming the correct diagnosis.

The symptom complex that defines food protein-induced enterocolitis syndrome is the result of a severe form of food allergy that is presumed to be

Mirna Chehade MD
Instructor, Pediatric Allergy/Immunology and Gastroenterology, Mount Sinai School of Medicine

Scott H. Sicherer MD (for correspondence)
Associate Professor of Pediatrics, Division of Allergy/Immunology, Mount Sinai School of Medicine,
Box #1198, One Gustave L. Levy Place, New York, NY 10029, USA
E-mail: scott.sicherer@mssm.edu

cell-mediated and is not generally associated with positive tests for 'food allergy' (*e.g.* IgE antibodies directed to the causal food protein). The syndrome is being described with increasing frequency and reactions are being identified to a broadening range of foods. The goal of this chapter is to improve the paediatrician's ability to identify and manage this disorder. We will discuss the clinical features, diagnosis, management and natural course of this potentially severe form of food allergy.

HISTORICAL PERSPECTIVE

In 1967, Gryboski[1] described a series of 21 infants hospitalised with diarrhoea starting at the age of 2 days to 4.5 months. Most of these infants had blood or mucus in their stools and were failing to thrive. Their symptoms resolved after substituting their cow's milk formula for a protein hydrolysate or a soy formula. In a subsequent report in 1978, Powell[2] described a series of 9 infants with protracted diarrhoea with occasional mucus or blood that started within 2 weeks of the infants' first feeding, and was associated with vomiting. These gastrointestinal symptoms occurred during feeding with a cow's milk based formula, and then resolved with substitution of a soy formula, only to recur 1–2 weeks later. Their symptoms resolved upon switching to a protein hydrolysate formula. Powell identified an adverse response related to the intact proteins through oral food challenges of these infants.

CLINICAL PRESENTATION

Food protein-induced enterocolitis syndrome is primarily a disorder of infants characterised by a symptom complex that includes non-specific symptoms of vomiting, diarrhoea (usually haem-positive), failure to thrive, and possibly dehydration and shock.[2-4] The prevalence of food protein-induced enterocolitis syndrome is not known. The pattern of symptoms differs depending upon the chronicity of ingestion of the causal food and results in two distinct patterns of illness.

TYPICAL SYMPTOMS WITH CHRONIC EXPOSURE TO THE CAUSAL PROTEIN

Infants with food protein-induced enterocolitis syndrome who are formula fed typically develop vomiting and diarrhoea which may be mucoid. Blood in the stools is often found, either gross or occult. Some infants present with vomiting and irritability before the onset of diarrhoea. Most infants are eventually noted to be malnourished and failing to thrive. If left untreated, dehydration, lethargy and shock may eventually occur. These chronic symptoms typically resolve upon switching to a protein hydrolysate formula.[2,3]

SYMPTOMS AFTER ACUTE RE-EXPOSURE TO THE CAUSAL PROTEIN

After a period of avoidance of the offending allergen, if these infants are later exposed to it, a violent reaction with a specific pattern may occur. Typically, 1–3 h after re-exposure to the offending allergen, there is onset of vomiting. Severe and repetitive vomiting is typical. These symptoms may, for about 20%

of those affected, lead to dehydration and hypotension. Laboratory evaluation during this reaction reveals elevated peripheral polymorphonuclear leukocyte counts, acidosis, and occasionally methaemoglobinaemia (cyanosis).[2-4] This clinical presentation appears similar to bacterial sepsis. Diarrhoea typically ensues within a few hours of ingestion of the protein and stool examination reveals the presence of blood and leukocytes, eosinophils and increased carbohydrates, reflecting small bowel involvement.[5] The symptom pattern noted on re-exposure after dietary avoidance is also typical of the pattern seen when food protein-induced enterocolitis syndrome is induced by solid foods, probably related to the manner in which solids are introduced (*e.g.* at occasional meals compared to milk or soy protein provided early on and frequently).[6]

CAUSATIVE FOOD PROTEINS

PROTEINS IN INFANT FORMULAE

Cow's milk protein introduced initially in the form of infant formula is the most common food to trigger food protein-induced enterocolitis syndrome. When infants are formula fed from birth, symptoms usually begin within the first 2–3 weeks of life. Initially, infants are noticed to have irritability, then severe vomiting and loose stools. The latter are occasionally mucoid, and have frank or occult blood.[5] Of those patients with cow's milk-associated food protein-induced enterocolitis syndrome, 50–60% will also have soy protein-associated food protein-induced enterocolitis syndrome.[3,7] There are food-allergic disorders associated with maternally ingested food proteins passed to the allergic infant in breast milk.[8-10] However, food protein-induced enterocolitis syndrome is not typically described to occur in exclusively breast-feeding infants.

SOLIDS

Proteins other than milk and soy, usually in the form of solid foods fed to infants, may trigger food protein-induced enterocolitis syndrome. In a report of 14 infants with food protein-induced enterocolitis syndrome provoked by solid foods, 78% were found to react to more than one food protein, and 64% also had symptoms to cow's milk and/or soy.[6] The causal foods were cereals (most commonly oat and rice) and less commonly vegetables and poultry meat. In contrast to the infants with milk/soy-induced food protein-induced enterocolitis syndrome, infants with symptoms to solid foods were older at symptom onset (median age, 5.5 months; range, 3–7 months) compared to 1 month (range, 2 days to 12 months) in cow's milk and/or soy food protein-induced enterocolitis syndrome. Food protein-induced enterocolitis syndrome induced by chicken, turkey, peas and lentils has also been described.[11]

PATHOPHYSIOLOGY

The more typical type of food-allergic reaction manifesting with acute hives, asthma and anaphylaxis is associated with IgE antibodies to the causal food proteins. In contrast, food protein-induced enterocolitis syndrome is not typically associated with detectable IgE antibodies. The symptoms are reproducible, related to specific proteins (and not all proteins) and induce evidence of an inflammatory response; therefore, food protein-induced enterocolitis syndrome is considered an allergy (adverse immune response). The presumption, considering the delayed onset of symptoms and chronic course, is that the immune mechanisms involved are due to a cell-mediated hypersensitivity to the food. This mechanism characterises a number of chronic allergic reactions that have an indolent clinical course.[12] Unfortunately, detailed investigations of the pathophysiology of food protein-induced enterocolitis syndrome are limited, because the diagnosis is clinical (hence biopsies are rarely performed) and there are limitations on the invasiveness of laboratory tests that can be performed for infants. Therefore, investigators have mainly focused on examining the peripheral blood mononuclear cells of these infants, namely their *in vitro* proliferative and secretory responses to the offending food protein.

INCREASE IN ANTIGEN-SPECIFIC LYMPHOCYTE PROLIFERATION AND 'PRO-INFLAMMATORY' CYTOKINE RESPONSES

Van Sickle and co-workers[13] demonstrated that *in vitro* stimulation of peripheral lymphocytes of infants with food protein-induced enterocolitis syndrome with the causal food protein resulted in greater cell proliferation than in controls. The enhanced lymphocyte responses were specific to the food proteins responsible for clinical symptoms, as determined by food challenges. To characterise further this immune reaction, several studies investigated cytokine production by lymphocytes in patients with delayed-type gastrointestinal reactions to food proteins, though not all of the patients studied fit strict criteria for food protein-induced enterocolitis syndrome. Hill *et al.*[14] demonstrated increased *in vitro* production of the pro-inflammatory cytokine interferon (IFN)-γ in response to β-lactoglobulin (a milk protein) stimulation of peripheral lymphocytes from patients with late reactions to cow's milk protein. Other investigators studied the secretion of another inflammatory cytokine, tumour necrosis factor-α (TNF-α), by peripheral lymphocytes when cultured in the presence of cow's milk protein. It was increased in infants with cow's milk allergy with intestinal symptoms, compared to those of infants who had recovered from cow's milk allergy.[15,16]

Cytokine responses in intestinal tissue have been investigated in a limited fashion. Chung *et al.*[17] examined TNF-α in duodenal biopsy specimens of infants with food protein-induced enterocolitis syndrome. They found it to be increased in those with villous atrophy compared to those without villous atrophy or controls. Other investigators demonstrated an increase of this cytokine in the stools after positive milk challenge in patients with cow's milk allergy and gastrointestinal manifestations.[18,19]

DECREASE IN REGULATORY, 'ANTI-INFLAMMATORY' CYTOKINE RESPONSES

Transforming growth factor-β (TGF-β) is an important cytokine involved in the development of oral tolerance to food proteins. This cytokine and its receptors were found to be lower in the duodenum of patients with food protein-induced enterocolitis syndrome than in controls.[17] However, these study results were limited because many patients studied had intestinal villous atrophy, and since TGF-β and one of its receptors were found mainly on villous epithelial cells, this finding could have been influenced by atrophy. Clearly, the immune mechanisms underlying food protein-induced enterocolitis syndrome are only partly understood.

ENDOSCOPIC AND HISTOLOGICAL FINDINGS

Endoscopy and biopsies are rarely undertaken in the evaluation of food protein-induced enterocolitis syndrome because the diagnosis is clinical and can be confirmed with oral food challenge. However, features of the biopsy results during active disease are known, but are unfortunately non-specific and non-diagnostic. In infants with frank rectal bleeding, changes in the colonic mucosa are found, ranging in severity from mild friability (easy bleeding with swabbing) or minute ulcers to severe spontaneous haemorrhage and large ulcers.[5] Rectal biopsy specimens demonstrate acute inflammatory cells within the lamina propria or in the wall of the rectal glands, with occasional crypt abscesses.[5,20] In addition to colitis, the majority of infants with food protein-induced enterocolitis syndrome have evidence of small bowel damage, with variable degrees of villous atrophy.[2] Clinically, this may present as carbohydrate malabsorption, with very watery stools that are positive for reducing substances.[5]

STOOL TESTS

Leukocytes are found in smears of stool mucus when stained with Hansel stain. In addition, a finding more specific to food protein-induced enterocolitis syndrome is eosinophils and eosinophilic debris, but Hansel's stain must be used, rather than Gram's stain or toluidine blue, which do not stain eosinophilic material.[5] Evidence of carbohydrate malabsorption may be found in some infants.[5]

ALLERGY TESTS

As indicated previously, this disorder is not typically associated with IgE antibody to the causal proteins and, therefore, allergy skin prick tests or serum tests for food-specific IgE antibody are typically negative.[3] However, a small subset of children with food protein-induced enterocolitis syndrome may, later in their course, show evidence of IgE antibody to causal foods.[3,6] Patch testing is a modality to determine delayed-type (cell-mediated) reactions to allergens. Test agents are applied to the skin for 24 h and the area is assessed 2 and 3 days later for signs of inflammation. The potential role of patch testing, which has been reported to be useful in diagnosing causative foods in atopic dermatitis,[21] is not yet studied in food protein-induced enterocolitis syndrome.

DIFFERENTIAL DIAGNOSIS

Many disorders cause symptoms that overlap those of food protein-induced enterocolitis syndrome. Consideration for infection has already been discussed.

The following discussion is not meant to be comprehensive but will review several common clinical problems that may be considered. If the main presenting symptom is haem-negative diarrhoea, congenital and malabsorptive conditions may be considered. If, on the other hand, the diarrhoea is haem-positive, different conditions causing colitis or enterocolitis are more likely. If vomiting is the dominant symptom, reflux needs to be considered. Finally, other allergic conditions with overlapping symptoms must be taken into account. We discuss here the different conditions and some clues that help differentiating them from food protein-induced enterocolitis syndrome.

NON-BLOODY DIARRHOEA

Congenital malabsorptive disorders that cause chronic diarrhoea include congenital microvillous atrophy, also referred to as microvillous inclusion disease, and tufting enteropathy. These manifest with diarrhoea, and their diagnosis can only be made upon electron microscopic examination of small intestinal biopsy sections.[22,23] Congenital chloridorrhea also presents with severe diarrhoea, and its diagnosis can be made by measuring stool electrolytes. Nutrient malabsorptive disorders such as congenital glucose and galactose malabsorption also present with severe diarrhoea resulting in failure to thrive. The stools test positive for reducing substances in these disorders.[24] In contrast to food protein-induced enterocolitis syndrome, all the above disorders are characterised by absence of mucosal inflammation. Therefore, stool tests for blood and leukocytes are useful to differentiate these disorders from food protein-induced enterocolitis syndrome.

BLOODY DIARRHOEA

Diarrhoea with minor rectal bleeding

Conditions that present with diarrhoea in infants where the stools are positive for occult blood and leukocytes include chronic postenteritis diarrhoea that may occur in older infants, and Hirschsprung's disease with resultant enterocolitis-induced diarrhoea. The latter condition should be suspected if the infant has had delayed passage of meconium during the first 24 h of life, or if constipation preceded the diarrhoea, and can be confirmed by a rectal suction biopsy.[25]

Diarrhoea with significant rectal bleeding

If rectal bleeding is a prominent feature of the diarrhoea, other conditions need to be considered, including necrotizing enterocolitis, which typically occurs in pre-term infants, although it may occur in term infants with congenital heart disease.[26] Stress ulcers or gastritis may cause occult rectal bleeding in the critically ill infants, and coagulopathies such as Von Willebrand's disease relatively frequently manifest with mucosal bleeding. Finally, intussusception needs to be considered in the older infant with colicky pain and irritability.[27]

INFECTIONS

Infections causing bloody diarrhoea should be considered. Causal organisms include enteric organisms, such as *Clostridium difficile* causing pseudomembranous

Table 1 Features of food protein-induced enterocolitis syndrome and other causes of colitis

Features in common
- Vomiting
- Bloody or guaiac positive diarrhoea
- Friability and/or ulcers on proctoscopy
- Stool mucus containing leukocytes (neutrophils and lymphocytes)
- Abnormal white blood cell count with predominance of neutrophils

Distinguishing features
- Absence of fever
- Longer prodrome
- Eosinophils and eosinophil debris in stool smears
- Carbohydrate malabsorption, suggestive of small bowel damage (suggestive feature)
- Failure to isolate a pathogen on stool culture (suggestive feature)
- Rapid disappearance (in 24–48 h) of blood and leukocytes from the stool after the offending antigen has been removed from the diet, without use of antibiotics (suggestive feature)

Adapted from Powell.[5]

enterocolitis, rotavirus, and non-enteric infections such as infection with Gram-negative bacteria. Septicaemia is often suspected in infants with food protein-induced enterocolitis syndrome upon presentation to their physician, prompting cultures of blood, urine and even cerebrospinal fluid. Table 1 outlines certain features that may help differentiate food protein-induced enterocolitis syndrome from other causes of colitis.

GASTRO-OESOPHAGEAL REFLUX DISEASE

When vomiting is the predominant feature, gastro-oesophageal reflux disease should be considered. Failure to thrive is rarely present in patients with gastro-oesophageal reflux, however, which helps to differentiate this entity from food protein-induced enterocolitis syndrome. Furthermore, failure to respond to anti-reflux measures should prompt consideration of a possibility of an allergy to milk, including food protein-induced enterocolitis syndrome.

ALLERGIC CONDITIONS OTHER THAN FOOD PROTEIN-INDUCED ENTEROCOLITIS SYNDROME

Other allergic disorders may also present with variable degrees of vomiting and/or diarrhoea. These gastrointestinal allergic disorders have specific features that help to distinguish them from food protein-induced enterocolitis syndrome.

Dietary protein-induced proctitis/proctocolitis

Infants with this disorder present with visible specks or streaks of blood mixed with mucus in the stool in the first few months of life. Cow's milk protein, and less commonly soy protein, are the common triggers.[28] In contrast to food protein-induced enterocolitis syndrome, most infants are symptomatic while they are breast-fed; the causal protein in the mother's diet is thought to be transmitted via breast milk.[8] Some infants are even symptomatic on a protein hydrolysate formula. Infants with this condition, however, do not have vomiting, diarrhoea or growth failure, which are typical of food protein-induced enterocolitis syndrome. Rectal biopsies from these infants reveal marked infiltration with eosinophils,[29] though such biopsy is usually not required for diagnosis because symptoms resolve within days of maternal elimination of the causal food protein.

Dietary protein enteropathy

Dietary protein enteropathy is characterised by protracted vomiting and diarrhoea, most commonly attributed to ingestion of cow's milk protein. Villus atrophy is the primary histological abnormality and protein loss with resulting oedema may occur. The symptoms overlap those of food protein-induced enterocolitis syndrome in many ways but are less dramatic, do not include colitis and no acute reactions occur when the food is taken intermittently.[30]

Eosinophilic gastroenteropathies

This group of disorders is characterised by eosinophilic inflammation of the gut. Specific symptoms vary by degree and location of inflammation. Manifestations of eosinophilic gastroenterocolitis may, like food protein-induced enterocolitis syndrome, include vomiting and diarrhoea; however, the onset of symptoms upon exposure to the causal food is slow. No dramatic reaction such as hypotension and shock occur (unless the patient has IgE antibodies to the food which may occur in this disorder).[12]

DIAGNOSIS

The diagnosis food protein-induced enterocolitis syndrome is typically delayed because of overlap of symptoms with sepsis; recurrent reactions are common.[6] Therefore, a suspicion for food protein-induced enterocolitis syndrome is the primary factor toward a successful clinical diagnosis. Criteria for a clinical diagnosis have been outlined by Powell[5] with some suggested modifications based upon later observations that the disorder is also caused by proteins other than milk/soy and can develop in older infants. Diagnosis should be sought with advice and consultation from physicians with specialty training in gastroenterology and/or allergy and experience with oral food challenges. A paediatric gastroenterologist may need to be consulted to help rule out other entities especially if the challenge results are negative or symptom patterns are unclear. Infants are diagnosed with 'typical' food protein-induced enterocolitis syndrome if they meet the following criteria:[3]

1. Onset of symptoms before 9 months of age.

2. Repeated exposure to the offending food elicits diarrhoea and/or repetitive vomiting within 24 h without any other cause of the symptoms.

3. No symptoms other than gastrointestinal are elicited by the offending food.

4. Removal of the offending protein from the diet results in resolution of the symptoms, and/or a standardised food challenge elicits diarrhoea and/or vomiting (outlined below).

A suggestion for a diagnostic category of 'atypical food protein-induced enterocolitis syndrome' has been made to account for reports of a slightly older age group that may be affected (up to 12 months) and rare patients with elevated IgE levels to the offending food who otherwise fulfil all of the typical criteria of food protein-induced enterocolitis syndrome including challenge.[31]

CHALLENGE

INDICATIONS FOR CHALLENGE

An oral challenge is undertaken by feeding the suspected food under physician observation with preparation to treat any reactions. An oral challenge to the suspected causal food is considered if the diagnosis is otherwise unclear from the initial history and symptom complex , or to determine if the child developed tolerance to the causative food protein. Considering the natural course of the allergy, oral challenges may be considered for the purpose of monitoring for resolution of the allergy about 12–24 months after the initial diagnosis assuming no inter-current reactions.[5,31] In some cases, challenges may be appropriate to 'high- risk' foods not yet ingested by patients with food protein-induced enterocolitis syndrome to another food;[6] for example, in a patient who reacted to milk and has not tried soy, or in a patient who reacted to oat and has not tried rice.

CHALLENGE PROTOCOL

Oral challenges for food protein-induced enterocolitis syndrome can result in hypotension and shock; therefore, challenges must me undertaken in facilities prepared to manage these eventualities (*e.g.* a hospital). The challenge should be administered by an experienced clinician with a full staff experienced in emergency resuscitation available with medications. Informed consent should be obtained and the utility of the challenge (*e.g.* relative importance of the result for nutritional/social reasons in relation to risk) should be discussed in detail.

Before the challenge is started, an intravenous line should be inserted. Emergency medications should be immediately available. Patients should remain under medical supervision for 6–8 h, regardless of the outcome of the challenge, and longer if the challenge was positive. When a challenge is positive, patients often require intravenous fluids and may need steroids.[3] A detailed discussion of the details of preparation for an oral food challenge are beyond the scope of this review, but have been published.[32]

The amount of protein given for challenge has been recommended at 0.6 g of protein per kg of body weight.[33] After noting reactions at lower doses, a lower total amount of protein (0.15–0.3 g protein per kg of body weight) was recently recommended if the infant has a history of a severe reaction after a small ingestion.[3] Tables 2 and 3 outline general steps for undertaking a monitored oral food challenge and criteria for interpretation. Reactions are

Table 2 Steps to be followed in a challenge protocol

Confirm weight gain and absence of gastrointestinal symptoms while not ingesting the causal protein
Obtain baseline stool sample for blood, leukocytes and eosinophils, and CBC with a differential
Place intravenous catheter
Prepare emergency medications (intravenous saline, epinephrine, steroids)
Administer challenge
Observe for symptoms (usual onset 1–4 h)
Repeat CBC at 6–8 h post-challenge
Collect subsequent stools for the next 24 h
Adapted from Powell.[5]

Table 3 Challenge

Criteria for a positive challenge 　　Symptoms: vomiting and/or diarrhoea not present before challenge 　　Fecal blood (gross or occult) not present before challenge 　　Fecal leukocytes not present before challenge 　　Fecal eosinophils not present before challenge 　　Increase in peripheral PMN count by > 3500 cells/mm^3
Positive challenge: 3 or more criteria met
Equivocal challenge: 2–5 criteria met
Negative challenge: 0–1 criterion met
Adapted from Powell.[5]

treated with fluid resuscitation (*e.g.* a bolus of normal saline) and possibly intravenous steroids to quell the presumed T cell-mediated response. Patients are kept under close observation and monitored until they are able to take fluids on their own and are haemodynamically stable. Additional therapies may be needed depending upon symptoms (*e.g.* vasopressors).

TREATMENT

The cornerstone of therapy for food protein-induced enterocolitis syndrome is strict avoidance of the causal food. No pharmacological therapies have been studied. In infants with cow's milk protein-induced disease, substitution of an extensive milk protein hydrolysate is generally recommended and usually tolerated. Soy is not generally recommended as a substitute formula because about 50% of patients react if they are allergic to cow's milk.[7,31] Partial hydrolysates would contain significant residual milk proteins and are not suggested. For the rare patient reactive to a protein hydrolysate due to persistence of peptide fragments in these formulas, an amino-acid formula is appropriate.[34] Families of infants with food protein-induced enterocolitis syndrome must be instructed about the careful avoidance of cow's milk and soy. Food labels should be read carefully and parents must be educated about proper identification of milk proteins (*e.g.* terms such as casein and whey). Parents must also be educated about issues of cross-contact among foods that could lead to the causal protein being present in particular meals. Lay organisations such as the Anaphylaxis Campaign (<www.anaphylaxis.org.uk>) in the UK and the Food Allergy & Anaphylaxis Network in the US (<www.foodallergy.org>) can be very helpful in assisting families with these issues.

In the event of an inadvertent exposure, patients should be instructed to seek medical attention promptly because reactions can include hypotension. Treatment could require therapies similar to those mentioned above for treatment of positive challenges. If a child with food protein-induced enterocolitis syndrome presents with symptoms, the treating physician must also consider additional potential causes of the noted symptoms (*e.g.* consider possibility of poisoning, infection, *etc.*).

NATURAL COURSE

Fortunately, patients with food protein-induced enterocolitis syndrome will likely outgrow their sensitivity after 12–24 months. Therefore, follow-up challenges may be considered at 12—24 monthly intervals.[3] The decision to perform the challenge, and the timing, may be adjusted depending upon the patient's specific history. For example, one may choose to wait longer when a small exposure caused a severe reaction compared to a history that indicates accidental exposure did not result in symptoms. While the disorder is not associated with IgE antibody to the foods, a small subset of patients have developed IgE to the causal foods and seem to be less likely to develop tolerance.[3] In addition, the patients who develop IgE antibodies to the eliminated foods have an increased risk to additionally experience respiratory or skin reactions and may require a different approach to evaluation for this risk (*e.g.* expectation of possible anaphylactic reactions).

CONCLUSIONS

Infantile food protein-induced enterocolitis syndrome should be considered in the infant with vomiting, diarrhoea and failure to thrive, as well as in the infant with a picture of septicaemia but negative cultures who has introduced a new food. Proper diagnosis and management of this condition are crucial to allow a healthy infancy until tolerance to the offending foods is achieved.

Key points for clinical practice

- Food protein-induced enterocolitis syndrome is a type of food allergy characterised by vomiting and diarrhoea in infants.
- Infants with food protein-induced enterocolitis syndrome who continue to ingest the causal food typically have failure to thrive.
- After avoidance of a causal food and resolution of symptoms, re-introduction may result in a sepsis-like picture with onset of profuse

(continued from previous page)

vomiting about 2 h after ingestion, then diarrhoea and possibly acidemia and shock.

- Diagnosis of food protein-induced enterocolitis syndrome is made clinically or by challenge with the causal food.
- Cow's milk is the most common causal protein.
- Most infants with food protein-induced enterocolitis syndrome and milk allergy are also reactive to soy.
- Some infants have food protein-induced enterocolitis syndrome from solid foods, typically oat and rice.
- IgE levels and prick skin tests to the offending foods are typically negative.
- Stools may have occult or gross blood, leukocytes and/or eosinophilic debris.
- Challenge with the causal protein should be done under medical supervision.
- Management of food protein-induced enterocolitis syndrome consists of eliminating the allergenic food from the diet.
- If cow's milk is the causal food, an extensive protein hydrolysate formula is recommended.
- If solid foods are the offending allergens, strict avoidance is required.
- Challenge with the causal protein may be done 12–24 months later to determine development of tolerance, but must be done under physician supervision under controlled settings to manage potentially severe reactions.

References

1. Gryboski JD. Gastrointestinal milk allergy in infants. *Pediatrics* 1967; **40**: 354–362.
2. Powell GK. Milk- and soy-induced enterocolitis of infancy. *J Pediatr* 1978; **93**: 553–560.
3. Sicherer SH, Eigenmann PA, Sampson HA. Clinical features of food protein-induced enterocolitis syndrome. *J Pediatr* 1998; **133**: 214–219.
4. Murray KF, Christie DL. Dietary protein intolerance in infants with transient methemoglobinemia and diarrhea. *J Pediatr* 1993; **122**: 90–92.
5. Powell GK. Food protein-induced enterocolitis of infancy: differential diagnosis and management. *Compr Ther* 1986; **12**: 28–37.
6. Nowak-Wegrzyn A, Sampson HA, Wood RA, Sicherer SH. Food protein-induced enterocolitis syndrome caused by solid food proteins. *Pediatrics* 2003; **111**: 829–835.
7. Burks AW, Casteel HB, Fiedorek SC, Williams LW, Pumphrey CL. Prospective oral food challenge study of two soybean protein isolates in patients with possible milk or soy protein enterocolitis. *Pediatr Allergy Immunol* 1994; **5**: 40–45.
8. Lake AM, Whitington PF, Hamilton SR. Dietary protein-induced colitis in breast-fed infants. *J Pediatr* 1982; **101**: 906–910.
9. Kilshaw PJ, Cant AJ. The passage of maternal dietary proteins into human breast milk. *Int Arch Allergy Appl Immunol* 1984; **75**: 8–15.
10. Makinen-Kiljunen S, Palosuo T. A sensitive enzyme-linked immunosorbent assay for determination of bovine β-lactoglobulin in infant feeding formulas and in human milk. *Allergy* 1992; **47**: 347–352.

11. Levy Y, Danon YL. Food protein-induced enterocolitis syndrome – not only due to cow's milk and soy. *Pediatr Allergy Immunol* 2003; **14**: 325–329.
12. Sampson HA. Update on food allergy. *J Allergy Clin Immunol* 2004; **113**: 805–813.
13. Van Sickle GJ, Powell GK, McDonald PJ, Goldblum RM. Milk- and soy protein-induced enterocolitis: evidence for lymphocyte sensitization to specific food proteins. *Gastroenterology* 1985; **88**: 1915–1921.
14. Hill DJ, Hosking CS, Wood PR. Gamma-interferon production in cow milk allergy. *Allergy* 1993; **48**: 75–80.
15. Heyman M, Darmon N, Dupont C *et al.* Mononuclear cells from infants allergic to cow's milk secrete tumor necrosis factor α, altering intestinal function. *Gastroenterology* 1994; **106**: 1514–1523.
16. Benlounes N, Candalh C, Matarazzo P, Dupont C, Heyman M. The time course of milk antigen-induced TNF-α secretion differs according to the clinical symptoms in children with cow's milk allergy. *J Allergy Clin Immunol* 1999; **104**: 863–869.
17. Chung HL, Hwang JB, Park JJ, Kim SG. Expression of transforming growth factor β1, transforming growth factor type I and II receptors, and TNF-α in the mucosa of the small intestine in infants with food protein-induced enterocolitis syndrome. *J Allergy Clin Immunol* 2002; **109**: 150–154.
18. Majamaa H, Miettinen A, Laine S, Isolauri E. Intestinal inflammation in children with atopic eczema: faecal eosinophil cationic protein and tumor necrosis factor-α as non-invasive indicators of food allergy. *Clin Exp Allergy* 1996; **26**: 181–187.
19. Kapel N, Matarazzo P, Haouchine D *et al.* Fecal tumor necrosis factor α, eosinophil cationic protein and IgE levels in infants with cow's milk allergy and gastrointestinal manifestations. *Clin Chem Lab Med* 1998; **37**: 29–32.
20. Halpin TC, Byrne WJ, Ament ME. Colitis, persistent diarrhea, and soy protein intolerance. *J Pediatr* 1977; **91**: 404–407.
21. Niggemann B, Reibel S, Wahn U. The atopy patch test (APT) – a useful tool for the diagnosis of food allergy in children with atopic dermatitis. *Allergy* 2000; **55**: 281–285.
22. Bell SW, Kerner JA, Sibley RK. Microvillous inclusion disease – the importance of electron microscopy for diagnosis. *Am J Surg Pathol* 1991; **15**: 1157–1164.
23. Reifen RM, Cutz E, Griffiths AM, Ngan BY, Sherman PM. Tufting enteropathy: a newly recognized clinicopathological entity associated with refractory diarrhea in infants. *J Pediatr Gastroenterol Nutr* 1994; **18**: 379–385.
24. Vanderhoof JA. Diarrhea. In: Wyllie R, Hyams JS. (eds) *Pediatric Gastrointestinal Disease: Pathophysiology, Diagnosis, Management.* Philadelphia, PA: W.B. Saunders, 1999; 32–42.
25. Dobbins WO, Bill AH. Diagnosis of Hirschsprung's disease excluded by rectal suction biopsy. *N Engl J Med* 1965; **272**: 990–993.
26. Polin RA, Pollack PF, Barlow B *et al.* Necrotizing enterocolitis in term infants. *J Pediatr* 1976; **89**: 460–462.
27. Heitlinger LA, McClung HJ. Gastrointestinal hemorrhage. In: Wyllie R, Hyams JS. (eds) *Pediatric Gastrointestinal Disease: Pathophysiology, Diagnosis, Management.* Philadelphia, PA: W.B. Saunders, 1999; 64–72.
28. Machida HM, Catto Smith AG, Gall DG, Trevenen C, Scott RB. Allergic colitis in infancy: clinical and pathological aspects. *J Pediatr Gastroenterol Nutr* 1994; **19**: 22–26.
29. Winter HS, Antonioli DA, Fukagawa N, Marcial M, Goldman H. Allergy-related proctocolitis in infants: diagnostic usefulness of rectal biopsy. *Mod Pathol* 1990; **3**: 5–10.
30. Kuitunen P, Visakorpi JK, Savilahti E, Pelkonen P. Malabsorption syndrome with cow's milk intolerance. Clinical findings and course in 54 cases. *Arch Dis Child* 1975; **50**: 351–356.
31. Sicherer SH. Food protein-induced enterocolitis syndrome: clinical perspectives. *J Pediatr Gastroenterol Nutr* 2000; **30**: S45–S49.
32. Bock SA, Sampson HA, Atkins FM *et al.* Double-blind, placebo-controlled food challenge (DBPCFC) as an office procedure: a manual. *J Allergy Clin Immunol* 1988; **82**: 986–997.
33. McDonald PJ, Goldblum RM, Van Sickle GJ, Powell GK. Food protein-induced enterocolitis: altered antibody response to ingested antigen. *Pediatr Res* 1984; **18**: 751–755.
34. Kelso JM, Sampson HA. Food protein-induced enterocolitis to casein hydrolysate formulas. *J Allergy Clin Immunol* 1993; **92**: 909–910.

Alistair J.A. Duff Alison K. Bliss

11

Reducing distress during venepuncture

Over the past 20 years, studies have shown that psychological techniques, when combined with appropriate anaesthesia, are highly effective in reducing the pain and fear associated with paediatric venepuncture. This chapter considers: (i) the developmental basis of perceptions and reactions to pain; (ii) aetiological factors of childhood fear; (iii) effective psychological and pharmacological interventions; and (iv) how clinicians can adapt and routinely use such techniques in everyday practice. Finally, it is argued that what is experienced clinically, is not 'needle-phobia' but procedural distress.

Many children and young people, who come to hospital, experience acute procedural pain, most commonly from venepuncture, intravenous (IV) cannulation, intramuscular (IM) and subcutaneous injections. Despite pharmacological advances, children continue to find these procedures the most frightening aspects of attending,[1] experiencing them as being unpredictable and outside of their control. Although tolerable for many, a large group do not cope well, resulting in a variety of negative emotional and behavioural difficulties including conditioned anxiety, emotional withdrawal, attempts to avoid or escape, and in some cases, severe tantrums or aggression.[2] All too often, the procedure is forsaken or restraint is applied, intensifying the misery for everyone involved.

Alistair J.A. Duff MA MSc DClinPsych (for correspondence)
Consultant Clinical Psychologist, Paediatric Psychology Services, Department of Clinical & Health Psychology, Ashley Wing Extension, St James's University Hospital, Leeds LS9 7TF, UK
E-mail alistair.duff@leedsth.nhs.uk

Alison K. Bliss MB ChB FRCA
Consultant Paediatric Anaesthetist, Children's Pain Service, Department of Anaesthetics, Lincoln Wing, St James's University Hospital, Leeds LS9 7TF, UK
E-mail alison.bliss@leedsth.nhs.uk

DEVELOPMENTAL UNDERSTANDING OF PAIN

Pain is not the single-modal entity it was once thought to be. On the contrary, it is a fluid and constantly evolving phenomenon, with multimodal physical, physiological, psychological and pathological components; the brain integrating nociceptive afferents, and other inputs and memories, to construct a continually evolving internal model. As understanding of the plasticity of the immature nervous system increases, it is apparent that the occurrence of iatrogenic pain and distress adversely affects the way these same insults are processed in the future, as the child matures.

NEUROBIOLOGY

Simple peripheral skin damage in immature animals causes increased nociceptive innervation of that area of skin, which remains long after wound healing and into adulthood.[3] Early exposure to painful stimuli also produces enduring changes in the opioid receptor pharmacology of the spinal cord. It is thought such changes may be diminished by adequate analgesia. This has been corroborated clinically, in studies demonstrating that, after painful stimuli months earlier, young babies exhibit an exaggerated pain response to painful stimuli occurring in a different body location.[4]

COGNITIVE DEVELOPMENT

Children's thinking not only changes as they develop but alters in specific and qualitative ways. Children's recollections of painful procedures, such as needle-insertion, are known to be vivid; however, these vary according to their cognitive abilities, in turn, affecting how pain is perceived, understood, remembered and reported (see Table 1).

Clinical practice needs to reflect both the increasing evidence on how the maturing nervous system can be physiologically altered by the pain and distress experienced, and the ways in which infants, children and young people cognitively and emotionally process such experiences, to ensure that procedures involving needle-insertion entail the minimum amount of pain and distress.

CHILDHOOD FEARS AND PHOBIAS

DEFINITION AND PREVALENCE

All children experience some level of fear as they grow up, this being age-appropriate, mild, adaptive and ephemeral, and typically arising from developing cognitive abilities in the presence of perceived threatening stimuli. In contrast, phobic fear is a response to a benign stimulus, which is out of proportion to the demands of the situation, cannot be explained, is beyond voluntary control and leads to avoidance.[6] Current diagnostic criteria for specific phobia continue to be based on these premises. Phobias are not highly prevalent in children and young people, with an average incidence of about 5% across studies.[7] They do, however, occur frequently and may result in considerable distress.

Table 1 Children and adolescents' understanding of pain and responses[5]

Age	Understanding & responses
0–3 months*	No apparent understanding of pain Memory for pain likely but not conclusively demonstrated Responses appear reflexive
3–6 months*	Response to pain supplemented with sadness and anger
6–18 months	Development of fear of painful situations Common words for pain evolve Loose localisation of pain
18–24 months	Use of the word 'hurt' to describe pain and non-cognitive coping strategies Awareness of methods of alleviating pain
24–36 months	Beginnings of pain description External causes attributed to pain Threat of immediate pain is overwhelming Future benefit not understood
36–60 months	Using more descriptive adjectives and attachment of associated emotions Difficulty in understanding that needle pain will be over quickly Spontaneous use of distraction
5–7 years	Clearer differentiation of levels of pain intensity Beginning to use cognitive coping strategies
7–11 years	Additional explanations of why pain hurts Concerns about pain limiting present activities rather than future ability
11+ years	Additional explanations of the value of pain Pain acknowledged as a 'feeling'

*It must be remembered that, contrary to previous beliefs, infants do feel pain.

NEEDLE PHOBIA OR ANTICIPATORY DISTRESS?

'Needle phobia' is a phrase which is often applied to children and young people who become so highly distressed during venepuncture that they have to be restrained or the procedure is abandoned. However, although the use of this term seems logical in light of current psychiatric taxonomy, there are fundamental flaws in applying such definitions to children and adolescents with such regularity. For example, when questioned, children neither view needles as 'benign stimuli', nor react in 'excessive'' or 'unreasonable' ways. Moreover, they rate their fear significantly higher *prior to* needle insertion[8] and react no differently when offered a needle-less venepuncture system.[9]

Whilst explaining the phenomenon medically or psychiatrically is superficially convenient (in that it is implied that blame is located 'within the patient'), it is of little value in reducing the frequency with which it occurs in paediatric contexts. On the contrary, what *is* commonly witnessed in the context of venepuncture is anticipatory or procedural distress. Consequently, there is as much need to revise the context and procedure, as there is to psychologically 'treat' the patient in whom such fear has arisen. This, however, does not explain why some children are able to tolerate needle-insertion and others are not.

AETIOLOGY

The term 'distress' relates to the complex interaction between pain, anxiety and fear. Contemporary explanations have attributed causation to interactions between individual, parental and situational factors. These have been extensively reviewed[10] and include the following:

Individual factors

1. **Genetic**. Inherited proneness is a controversial notion. Although there is no evidence of heritability for children with specific phobias, it is thought that specific fears and phobias have the lowest heritable estimates and the highest environmental influences.[11]

2. **Temperament**. Phobic anxiety and fear is significantly higher in 'inhibited' than in 'uninhibited' children.[7] Furthermore, children rated by their parents as active, intense or negative in mood, display higher levels of distress. Such temperament characteristics are known to determine whether a child is 'prepared' (*e.g.* told in advance), for venepuncture or not by their parents and the length of time they are left to tolerate attempts to insert a needle before abandonment, sedation or restraint.[12]

3. **Age and sex**. Pain and fear associated with needle-insertion decrease with age. In children over 8 years, girls rate needles as 'unpleasant' as opposed to 'intensely painful', more than boys.[13]

4. **General behaviour**. Externalising behaviours positively correlate with behavioural distress before, during and after needle-insertions. This suggests that a valid parent-report measure of childhood behaviour problems could be used in combination with other factors to predict those children at greatest risk for severe distress during venepuncture.[14]

5. **Experience**. Although there is no known relationship between the number of procedures involving needle-insertion and distress, the more negative the experience, the greater the subsequent anxiety, distress and non-cooperation.[15] In one study, over 60% of 7–18-year-olds remembered having experienced a very unpleasant and painful venepuncture.[8]

Parental factors

1. Parents of 'inhibited' children have a greater prevalence of phobias[16] raising the possibility of a familial (if not a genetic) link, which predisposes their child to heightened levels of general fearfulness and anxiety sensitivity.[7]

2. The relationship between parental anxiety and childhood distress during venepuncture is strong[17] and parents tend to be aware of this.[8]

3. Most parents prefer to be present during the procedure[8,18] and children believe this to 'help the most'.[19]

Situational factors

1. The environment and context within which venepuncture takes place influences levels of distress. Distinction needs to be drawn between those

who present acutely unwell, those who are more stable but who have little familiarity with attending hospital and those who have chronic conditions and frequent visits. Children in the former two groups have been reported to find needle-insertion more distressing than those in the latter.[20]

2. Children with recently diagnosed chronic conditions record higher ratings of pain and fear than those with longer histories.

3. Prolonged exposure to venepuncture 'cues' (*e.g.* seeing medical equipment and blood samples or hearing other children in distress) can also heighten fear unnecessarily. In many consultations, venepuncture is typically undertaken last, prolonging the period of anticipation.

PHARMACOLOGICAL INTERVENTIONS

Topical anaesthesia of the skin can be achieved by either direct physical (ethyl chloride, ice), or pharmacological (local anaesthetic) inhibition of nerve transmission. Topical anaesthetics form the basis of treatment and can be used alone or in combination with systemic agents and non-pharmacological interventions. The current range of topical and systemic agents affords clinicians the ability to alleviate pain and distress, safely and appropriately, in virtually all clinical situations.

TOPICAL AGENTS

Local anaesthetic penetration of the epidermis can be enhanced by using highly lipophilic drugs (tetracaine), high concentrations (EMLA®, eutectic mixture of local anaesthetics), or iontophoresis. Creams and gels require prolonged application under occlusive dressings but produce reliable and effective analgesia. Ethyl chloride spray is fast acting and has been shown to be comparable with EMLA® cream for use in peripheral intravenous cannulation in children (Table 2).

Iontophoresis, although less commonly used in the UK, has the advantage of faster onset times. With some iontophoretic preparations, the amount of drug delivered is directly proportional to the total electric charge applied (*i.e.* current [mA] x time [min] expressed in milliampere minutes [mAmin]). Children and adults receive the same dose but if the child experiences any discomfort during treatment or finds the electrical sensation unpleasant, the current level can be reduced and applied over a longer period

SYSTEMIC AGENTS

For some children, the distress associated with needle-insertion is such that topical anaesthesia and psychological treatment in combination, will not suffice, and systemic sedative or anxiolytic agents are required for urgent procedures requiring needle or cannula insertion (Table 3).

Many sedative agents produce only lack of awareness, not lack of pain, and therefore where possible, should be combined with topical (preferably), or systemic, analgesia. The ideal agent has a rapid onset, short duration, good side-effect profile and low risk of adverse events. Sucrose exhibits all of these properties

Table 2 Topical pharmacological interventions

Intervention	Age	Timescale	Mode of action	Advantages	Disadvantages
Ethyl chloride spray (Cryogesic®)	No age limit documented	Spray for 5–10 s for adequate analgesia	A volatile liquid Evaporates instantly when sprayed onto the skin, causing cooling to below 10°C Transmission of nerve impulses inhibited at such temperatures Adjacent skin protected from cooling effects by applying petroleum jelly	No advance preparation Few 'cues'	Rapid effect Unpleasant cold sensation from activation of adjacent sensory nerve endings (older children report as cold and numb sensations) Peripheral vasoconstriction in response to cold Reports of solvent abuse* Flammability
Lignocaine gel Iontophoresis ('Numby Stuff®', Northstar Iontophoretic Patch)	All Variety of patch sizes and drug concentrations	Effective anaesthesia of the skin (depth 10 mm) within 10 min	Iontophoresis is a drug delivery method that uses a small external electric current to deliver water-soluble, charged drugs into the skin Iontophoresis patches are adhesive gel-filled electrodes which contain lignocaine 2–4% with dilute concentrations of adrenaline Electrodes connected to a small battery-powered generator	No messy creams Few 'cues' Rapid effect	Iontophoresis of lignocaine with adrenaline can cause temporary blanching of the skin followed by transient erythema but process well-tolerated with few side effects
4% Tetracaine gel (Ametop)	> 1 month	Venepuncture 30 min Cannulation 45 min Apply for not more than 1 h Anaesthesia lasts 4–6 h	Highly lipophilic Easily crosses the stratum corneum of the epidermis to penetrate the underlying dermis and peripheral nerves	Vasodilator	Can cause localised erythema
EMLA® (eutectic mixture of local anaesthetics)	> 1 year Safe use in most neonates reported	Effective after 1 h Peak effect occurs after 90 min secondary to a depot effect Safe for up to 5 h	2.5% Lignocaine and 2.5% Prilocaine as an oil-water emulsion The concentration of drug in the droplets of the emulsion is so high (80%) that the stratum corneum is effectively penetrated	Can cause vasodilatation after vasoconstriction (biphasic action)	Vasoconstriction and blanching Prilocaine can lead to methaemaglobinaemia in neonates

*Leading to confusion, hallucinations, ataxia, short-term memory impairment, cardiac dysrhythmias, respiratory arrest and death.

Table 3 Systemic pharmacological interventions

Intervention	Age	Timescale	Mode of action	Advantages	Disadvantages
66% Sucrose	<34 weeks PCA 2 ml >34 weeks 4 ml	Give immediately prior to the procedure	Stimulate receptors in tongue, which activate opioid receptors in pain pathways. Effects reversed by naloxone. Analgesic effect enhanced with use of pacifier	No known side effects	Less effective in older babies
Inhaled nitrous oxide (Entonox®, Equanox®)	Babies up to 4 months. Requires co-operation by the child. Possible use in those > 3 years	Effective analgesia within 2 min	Available in pre-mixed cylinders as 50:50 mix of nitrous oxide and oxygen. Self-administered via: * inspiration-activated valve, * face or nasal mask, * mouth piece (less fearful for children and easier to use). Exact mechanism unknown. May involve opiate receptors as the analgesic action diminished by naloxone administration	Provides mild sedation with significant analgesia. Rapid onset. Brief duration	Contra-indications: • pneumothorax • bowel obstruction • recent cranial trauma • chronic respiratory disease. Staff must be trained and gas scavenged or area must be well-ventilated to ensure environmental levels below 100 ppm (HSE EH40). Can also cause unpleasant dizzy feelings, nausea and vomiting
Intranasal diamorphine 0.1 mg/kg to max 5 mg in 0.2 ml	Used down to 10 kg (~1 year)	Onset within 5 min. Duration 3–4 h	Nasal mucosa is highly vascular with a fenestrated epithelium so the small volume is totally absorbed instantly. First metabolite, monoacetylmorphine readily crosses blood-brain barrier to produce rapid analgesia	Rapid onset of systemic analgesia. Particularly useful in acute trauma situations where child is already in pain and distress from injury	Dissociation from pain. Contra-indications: • acute respiratory depression • raised ICP • head injury
Transmucosal fentanyl (Oralet, Actique) 10–15 mic/kg	Used down to 10 kg	Effective analgesia within 15–30 min of sucking lozenge	Highly lipid soluble opiate absorbed via oropharangeal mucosa and gastrointestinal absorption	Sweet-tasting palatable lozenge on a stick ('lollipop')	Over-sedation, pruritis, nausea and vomiting documented. Sedation not always associated with increased co-operation

but its effects are limited to neonates and those under 4 months old.[21] Advances in novel and painless methods of drug delivery have allowed the use of the opiates fentanyl and diamorphine. Although neither are free of side effects or adverse events, both produce sedation that will exceed the duration of almost all procedures involving needle insertion.

Recent UK guidelines for sedating children recommend the use of single sedative agents, as combinations are often associated with deeper levels of sedation and adverse effects.[22] In particular, it identifies inhaled nitrous oxide as a useful solo agent for sedation for painful procedures, as it produces rapid, but brief, sedation and analgesia. The use of other systemic agents for the provision of safe and effective 'conscious sedation' in children has recently been comprehensively reviewed.[23]

PSYCHOLOGICAL INTERVENTIONS

Behavioural and cognitive-behavioural interventions vary widely but mostly involve a combination of: progressive muscle relaxation training, guided imagery, distraction, modelling, and graded exposure and reinforcement scheduling. These are a variation on the influential studies of Elliot, Jay, Olsen and colleagues.[24,25] Using such techniques in association with injections, routine immunisations and venepuncture, consistently results in less pain and distress for children and young people.[26] These are now classified as 'well-established' treatments for paediatric procedure-related pain.[27]

RELAXATION TRAINING

This involves teaching the child how to gain control over symptoms of physiological arousal by breathing slowly and deeply, and releasing muscle tension. Several different types of relaxation are used in helping children gain mastery over procedural distress including: brief-relaxation (a brief exercise in which deep breathing is used to trigger relaxation throughout the body), tension-relaxation (requiring alternate tensing and relaxing of muscle groups), often combined with suggestion-method (e.g., auto-suggestions of feeling 'warm', 'relaxed' and 'heavy' are made).

GUIDED IMAGERY

Guided imagery typically accompanies relaxation training, where the child or young person is encouraged to bring to mind pleasant imagery and/or engage in fantasy 'scenes'. In addition, guided imagery is often used as cognitive distraction from any unpleasant thoughts associated with the procedure.

DISTRACTION

Distraction is commonly practiced but requires active participation and additional help from a parent, play specialist or nurse. (Trying to implement this and perform needle-insertion at the same time, only results in the child or young person focusing on the health carer and consequently the needle.) However, studies report mixed findings, with no compelling consensus emerging as to the most effective techniques to employ with children of specific ages.[14] Those that are developmentally appropriate and have been found to be successful[14,26] are listed in Table 4.

Table 4 Age-appropriate effective distraction techniques for children[a]

Group	Technique		
[Age]	Sensory	Physical	Cognitive
Infants 0–12 months	Gentle heat (e.g. warm blanket)[b] Snoezelon	Swaddling Appropriate massage[c] Oral pacifiers with/without Oral glucose/sucrose Rocking Positive touch Snoezelon	Visual stimulation (e.g. blowing bubbles) Auditory stimulation (e.g. music, singing) Snoezelon
Toddlers 13–24 months	As above Cold (e.g. ice-cubes applied to site of intended venepuncture)[b] Counter-irritation[b]	Appropriate positioning Sitting on parent's lap Hugging/holding Appropriate massage[c]	As above Action rhymes Kaleidoscopes Pop-up book Party blowers Mummy's jewellery
Pre-school 2–4 years	As above	As above Deep breathing Drawing[d] Electronic/'smart' toys[d] Brief relaxation	As above Counting, being read stories Non-medical conversation Video-taped cartoons Movies[e]
Young children 5–7 years	As above	Hand-held computers[d]	Guided imagery Engagement in fantasy scenes Thought stopping
Older children 8–11 years	As above	Video games[d]	As above

[a]Save materials most likely to distract for the procedure itself.
[b]Under the directions of physician.
[c]To be used with caution.
[d]Where procedures allows.
[e]Some evidence that nurse-coaching and film-distraction significantly increases child coping and reduces distress.

Note: Techniques often used in conjunction with parental prompts/rewards for using the distraction activity.
For children > 4 years, parental coaching may increase child's use of distraction.

MODELLING

Modelling is based on the principle that watching another child (preferably of the same sex, ethnicity and age group), displaying some anxiety about needle-insertion but overcoming it, will help the observer to utilise successful coping skills too. Modelling has been used in studies of reducing needle-related distress, but rarely in routine paediatric settings. However, advances in computer technology mean that large numbers of film clips can be easily accessed in busy clinics, (e.g. via CD-ROM and interactive computer games[28]). More commonly, modelling techniques are used to teach parents how to distract, and interact with their child during venepuncture.[20]

GRADED EXPOSURE AND REINFORCEMENT SCHEDULING

Graded exposure to the insertion of needles involves creating a hierarchy of successive approximations of the procedure (*e.g.* drawings of cannulae, removing packaging, cannulae being held up to arms with sleeves down), quickly building up to full behavioural rehearsals in a treatment room. Health carers (*e.g.* play specialists or psychologists), who are not capable of undertaking venepuncture, can help children reach the latter stage quickly; a task made easier by the child's knowledge that needle insertion cannot take place with this person. Consequently, qualified clinicians need to become co-workers as early in the hierarchy as possible. Reinforcement scheduling is an important part of graded exposure, whereby each accomplishment in the hierarchy is rewarded appropriately. It is important that token rewards are supplemented with abundant verbal praise from parents and professionals alike, this remaining in place once the reward has been withdrawn.

OTHER TECHNIQUES

Snoezelon is a multisensory area with equipment to create a dynamic environment offering stimulating input (auditory, visual, olfactory and tactile). Experiences are arranged to stimulate the primary senses without the need for intellectual activity, thus facilitating relaxation. The gentle stimulation has a soothing effect that helps to relieve agitation. Where available, this may help infants and pre-schoolers become calm prior to or following venepuncture.

The application of a very cold substance (*e.g.* ice on the skin) will produce local anaesthesia by directly inhibiting nerve transmission. As this is quickly and easily done without more formal 'medical' intervention (*e.g.* using creams and dressings), it may be better tolerated in children with high anxiety about medical settings or professionals, as well as the entire procedure. However, it does produce a cold sensation in adjacent skin that some children find unpleasant.

JOINT PHARMACOLOGICAL AND PSYCHOLOGICAL INTERVENTION

Topical anaesthesia should always be the basic component in addressing pain associated with needle insertion and cannulation. Psychological techniques are highly effective, relatively inexpensive and being increasing undertaken by a range of appropriately skilled professionals working in paediatric settings. Yet, neither psychology nor pharmacology can effectively address procedural distress. There is consistent evidence that combining empirically effective cognitive–behavioural approaches and topical anaesthesia, further reduces children's and young people's distress,[29–31] particularly during IM and IV needle or cannula insertion.

PROTOCOLS

Some hospitals have taken the step of developing protocols for the management of procedural distress. Whilst the main focus has been on the implementation of effective anaesthesia and psychological techniques, consideration has also been given to: (i) how often clinicians should attempt needle-insertion; (ii) balancing the training needs of junior doctors in terms of them gaining experience of needle and cannula insertion, with those of children known to be very fearful and (iii) the variety of settings where such procedures will be undertaken (*e.g.* A&E, wards and out-of-hours).

Reviews, guidelines and protocols have given consideration as to how services can be re-organised to incorporate non-pharmacological and psychological techniques routinely.[26,32] In all cases, the main concentration has been on prevention and minimising needle-related distress.

One other area of focus in protocols is on that of restraint or 'holding', *i.e.* the 'pro-active immobilisation of a part of the body to which a procedure is being carried out'.[33] Whilst at times it may be necessary to hold a child against their wishes in order to undertake urgent needle insertion, this needs to be balanced with issues of legality, consent, responsibility and risk management. Holding needs to take place in a safe and controlled way, by appropriately trained staff and only after all other alternatives have been exhausted.[33] One example of this is 'Positive Touch', a containment hold used for babies, one hand on head and one hand on trunk, and continued throughout the procedure.

PREVENTION

ASSESSMENT

Establishing how a child has previously reacted to needle insertion should become a routine part of assessment. If this has been negative, exact details of these experiences need to attained. (What happened? How did the child/young person react? At what point in the procedure did they become frightened?) Appropriate use (or in some cases, non-use) of topical anaesthesia can then be considered (*e.g.* if the child is likely to react emotionally to the application of EMLA® as an early warning signal that needle-insertion is imminent).

Assessment should also include a physical examination of the child. If venepuncture is likely to be technically difficult (*e.g.* no visible peripheral veins, multiple previous attempts with or without bruising), the clinician needs to consider if their skills and experience will be up to the task of a swift and painless first attempt success.

PREPARING AND UNDERTAKING

Non-pharmacological and psychological techniques can be easily incorporated into needle insertion. Some will be applicable to all children and young people; others will only apply if they become fearful and distressed. These are summarised in Table 5.

Mark out all peripheral veins suitable to the job and apply topical anaesthesia to all if possible. Failed cannulation that is pain-free has a better chance of continued tolerance of subsequent attempts. However, it is important to state that only one site will be used to stem any mis-perceptions that young children in particular may harbour, that there will be more than one needle insertion. Adequate exposure is critical to the effectiveness of topical anaesthesia; trying to rush it will lead to 'cream failure'. This may initiate the belief that venepuncture will always be painful, leading to loss of faith in communication with doctors and a refusal to try topical analgesia in the future.

Table 5 Preparation and procedure

Setting	Child/young person	Parents
PREPARATION Undertake in a designated treatment room, leaving the child in-patient 'space' or out-patient consulting room, as a 'safe place'	Build rapport and talk with child or young person in a non-treatment room	Actively encourage to stay; except if parent is also known to be fearful. If so, it may be useful for another relative/friend to be with the child during the procedure
Prepare the room • Ensure it is warm with adequate lighting • Minimise number of people • Have equipment ready in advance • Have distraction materials to hand	Include both the sensory and experiential aspects of the procedure	Needs to include both the sensory and experiential aspects.
	Give explanations about the procedure and levels of expected pain. This can address misconceptions, particularly those held by young children, who may need help in understanding that only the tip of the needle is inserted	Give explanations about needle or cannula insertion
Minimise disruptions • Switch pagers/phones to 'quiet' • Put 'engaged' signs on doors	Use a video-clip modelling the procedure if necessary	Prepare a leaflet for parents outlining 'what to do during your child's venepuncture'
Minimise venepuncture cues (e.g. keeping equipment out of sight)	Apply topical anaesthesia as appropriate allowing sufficient time for effectiveness	
PROCEDURE Where feasible venepuncture should take place as early in the consultation process as possible	Give permission to make a noise/cry	Give or repeat explicit instructions about their role during the procedure • Sit close to child or hold/sit the child on lap • Comfort/soothe child • Use/coach distraction • Not to give false reassurances (e.g. 'it won't hurt')
Avoid using loud voices or making startling noises	Give choices where appropriate • Site of insertion? • To look or not? Participation, with emphasis on collaboration, is important • Removing EMLA 'plasters' • Unwrapping equipment • Cleaning insertion site	
Carefully remove patches/tape from skin		
Undertake the procedure slowly, giving the child options to halt it if they start to feel frightened	Encourage utilisation of 'rehearsed skills' • Breathing exercises/relaxation • Guided imagery/distraction	
Restraint should only be applied after all alternative techniques have been tried		Negotiate in advance, if parents are to participate in restraint should it be required

Of course, when children and young people attend hospital regularly, time to undertake these steps may be more available. However, in acute or emergency situations where time is limited or pressured, it may be sufficient to only include some of these techniques, or indeed certain aspects of each. Nonetheless, in anticipation of needle-insertion, as a bare minimum it would be important to: (i) assess prior experience and utilisation of coping strategies; (ii) ensure that the procedure occurs as early as possible; (iii) give sensory and procedural information, and realistic expectations of pain-levels to both patient and parents; (iv) have as wide a range of distraction materials in the room as possible; (v) encourage parents to participate (to be there as an emotional resource); and (vi) give the child permission to cry or make a noise.

PROMISING NEW INTERVENTIONS

VIRTUAL REALITY AS DISTRACTION

To be effective, distraction must involve active processing and motor responses and substantially compete with the child or young person's attention to potentially distressing medical stimuli.[14] Therefore, using computer-generated visual recreations, which are engaging, interactive and stimulating, seems an ideal choice of distraction method. Early results have been encouraging with reductions in heart rate during dental procedures[34] and subjective ratings of pain during burn-wound management[35] being reported.

MEMORY REFRAMING

This novel cognitive intervention[36] utilised techniques that helped children and young people 'reframe' their recollections of lumbar puncture, encouraging them to: reconsider their reactions, recall the coping strategies they used and their effectiveness, and evaluate the extent of their distress. After giving feedback on the accuracy of reflections, participants were then given a visually striking card on which they wrote down their memories. The card was then used in subsequent treatments as a prompt. There were immediate reductions in anticipatory distress and subsequent reductions in procedural distress, with moderate to large effect sizes.

EYE MOVEMENT DESENSITISATION AND REPROCESSING (EMDR)

EMDR uses interruptions to saccadic eye movement to reduce visual intrusiveness associated with traumatic experiences and ensuing anxiety. Originally used to treat post-traumatic stress disorder, the utilisation of this intervention has been extended to try to reduce specific fears. Following EMDR in adults with needle-related distress, decreases in fear ratings were observed.[37] EMDR can be used with children over 8 years old but, as yet, evaluation remains absent.

COUNTER IRRITATION

Lately, there has been renewed interest in the clinical application of the 'gate theory of pain' to alleviate short-lived procedural pain. A-β sensory input (touch), from the scratch 'closes the gate' in the substantia gelatinosa of the dorsal horn to modulate nociceptive A δ and C input (pain), from the needle insertion, both directly and by increased descending inhibition. The technique of counter-irritation[38] is used as follows: (i) **stimulus**: firm rub or gentle scratching – a better technique, causing less tissue distortion; (ii) **site**: close to the puncture point but not too near the cannula tip, for example just outside the area of the dressing; and (iii) **time-scale**: beginning 1–2 s beforehand and continuing throughout the procedure.

NEEDLE-LESS INJECTORS

Needle-free gas powered injection systems are now being trialled and used with some success. Compressed gas within the syringe is used to create a pressurised stream of drug, which leaves the syringe through a micro-orifice to penetrate the skin up to a depth of 8 mm within a fraction of a second. Jet injectors can be used to deliver intradermal local anaesthetic immediately prior to venepuncture or cannulation when there is insufficient time for topical anaesthesia by cream or gel. Although they may be psychologically less traumatic, the delivery of drug by jet injector is not pain-free in itself, although it is significantly less painful than intradermal infiltration using a 25-G needle. Cannulation, however, may be more painful as the power of the jet distributes the drug over a wider area than that delivered by a 25-G needle and so the quality of local anaesthesia at the site of insertion may be diminished. It may also be more difficult following use of the injector, secondary to tissue distortion. The use of the injector appears to be more effective in those areas of the body with more subcutaneous tissue (*e.g.* children's hands and forearms), which supports their use as an aid to paediatric venepuncture.[39]

WAVE TECHNOLOGY, DRUG REPLACEMENT AND ANALGESIA

Advances in imaging technology are driving developments to use micro-, photo-, and magnetic-energy wave forms to enable specific changes at a molecular level in receptors, to prevent nerve conduction without the need for pharmacological agents. Work is now concentrating on the search for the best energy source and characteristics to provide anaesthesia or analgesia via computer-focused physical activation of receptor sites, with non-invasive external wave forms.[40]

CONCLUSIONS

Children and young people continue to find needle insertion one of the most frightening parts of attending hospital. Such fear needs to be placed within the context of the procedure and not simply seen as a 'psychiatric/phobic' problem within the child. As such, there is an onus on the medical and allied professions to revise such procedures to incorporate pharmacological and non-pharma-cological techniques, which are known to be successful in reducing associated pain and distress. Much is known about the usefulness of cognitive and behavioural techniques but clinical effectiveness will depend on how these are incorporated routinely.

Minimising physical and psychological distress during venepuncture is the responsibility of all concerned. Undertaking preparatory and procedural psychological approaches is something many health care professionals working in paediatric settings are skilled in. Support of lead clinicians, hospital guideline committees and parents is vital too, with large general paediatric out-patient clinics needing to be reviewed and restructured to some degree.

Current research is beginning to focus on practical screening tools to identify those children who may be at risk of experiencing distress associated with needle and cannula insertion (*e.g.* the use of child behaviour checklists). However, further studies need to continue to focus on which intervention strategies work for whom and in what settings and how benefits can be maintained in the longer term.

Key points for clinical practice – the 6 'P's

Prior knowledge

- Assess previous experience of needle/cannula insertion.
- Consider possible technical difficulties (*e.g.* poor venous access).
- Explore previous coping strategies.

Preparation

- Prepare the treatment room, having as much ready in advance as possible. Minimise disruptions and venepuncture 'cues'.
- Build rapport with children and prepare them psychologically, including both sensory and behavioural aspects of the procedure. Use filmed models if required.
- Actively encourage parents to stay. Prepare them about the sensory and physical aspects of the procedure and negotiate 'holding' responsibilities in advance.
- Try to undertake needle insertion as soon as possible in the consultation process (thus minimising exposure to 'cues').

Pharmacology

- Topical anaesthesia by temperature or local anaesthetic drug should always be the basic component of treatment to which psychological techniques with or without systemic agents are added.
- Always allow sufficient time for the topical anaesthetic to work before attempting the procedure.
- Even though they cannot express their distress, pain relief for neonates is important. Humanistic issues aside, it may prevent changes in the peripheral and central nervous systems in response to iatrogenic procedural pain.

Participation

- Involve the child as much as possible (*e.g.* choice of site, peeling of dressings, whether to look or not) and encourage utilisation of rehearsed skills (*e.g.* deep-breathing, relaxation, distraction).
- Give/repeat clear instructions about parents' roles in the procedure (*e.g.* sitting close to, and soothing, their child, coaching techniques).

Permission to make a noise

- Give permission for the child to make a noise. Sometimes actively planning this in advance becomes a distractor during needle/cannula insertion.

Patience

- Undertake the procedure slowly, giving the child options to halt it if they become very frightened.

References

1. Schechter NL, Blankson V, Pachter LM, Sullivan CM, Costa L. The ouchless place: no pain, children's gain. *Pediatrics* 1997; **99**: 890–894.
2. Blount RL, Landolf-Fritsche B, Powers SW, Sturges JW. Differences between high and low coping children and between parent and staff behaviors during painful medical procedures. *J Pediatr Psychol* 1991; **16**: 795–809.
3. Reynolds ML, Fitzgerald M. Long-term sensory hyperinnervation following neonatal skin wounds. *J Comp Neurol* 1995; **358**: 487–498.
4. Taddio A, Goldbach M, Ipp M, Stevens B, Koren G. Effect of neonatal circumcision on pain responses during vaccination in boys. *Lancet* 1995; **345**: 291–292.
5. McGrath PJ. Aspects of pain children and adolescents. *J Child Psychol Psychiatry* 1995; **36**: 717–730.
6. Marks IM. *Fears and Phobias*. New York: Academic Press, 1969.
7. Ollendick TH, King NJ, Muris P. Fears and phobias in children: phenomenology, epidemiology and aetiology. *Child Adolesc Mental Health* 2002; **7**: 98–106.
8. Duff AJA, Brownlee KG. The management of emotional distress during venepuncture. *Netherlands J Med* 1999; **54(Suppl)**: S8.
9. Polillo AM, Kiley J. Does a needleless injection system reduce anxiety in children receiving intramuscular injections? *Pediatr Nurs* 1997; **23**: 46–49.
10. Muris P, Merckelbach H. The etiology of childhood specific phobia: a multifactorial model. In: Vasey MW, Dodds MR. (eds) *The Developmental Psychopathology of Anxiety*. New York: OUP, 2000; 355–385.
11. Kendler KS, Neale MC, Kessler RC, Heath AC, Eaves LJ. The genetic epidemiology of phobias in women: the interrelationship of agoraphobia, social phobia and simple phobia. *Arch Gen Psychiatry* 1992; **49**: 273–281.
12. Lee LW, White-Traut RC. The role of temperament in pediatric pain response. Issues Comprehens Pediatr Nurs 1996; **19**: 49–63.
13. Goodenough B, Thomas W, Champion GD et al. Unravelling age effects and sex differences in needle pain; ratings of sensory intensity and unpleasantness of venepuncture pain by children and their parents. Pain 1999; **80**: 179–190.
14. Slifer KJ, Tucker CL, Dahlquist LM. Helping children and caregivers cope with repeated invasive procedures: how are we doing? J Clin Psychol Med Settings 2002; **9**: 131–152.
15. Dalquist LM, Gil KM, Armstrong FD, DeLawyer DD, Greene P, Wouori D. Preparing children for medical examinations: the importance of previous medical experience. Health Psychol 1986; **5**: 249–259.
16. Hirshfield DR, Rosenbaum JF, Biederman J et al. Stable behavioural inhibition and its association with anxiety disorder. J Am Acad Child Adolesc Psychiatry 1992; **31**: 103–111.
17. Jay SM, Ozolins M, Elliott CH, Caldwell S. Assessment of children's distress during painful medical procedures. Health Psychol 1983; **2**: 133–147.
18. Bauchner H, Vinci R, Waring C. Pediatric procedures: do parents want to watch? Pediatrics 1989; **84**: 907–909.
19. Ross DM, Ross SA. Childhood pain: the school-aged child's viewpoint. Pain 1984; **20**: 179–191.
20. Bauchner H, Vinci R, May A. Teaching parents how to comfort their children during common medical procedures. Arch Dis Child 1994; **70**: 548–550.
21. Stevens B, Yamada J, Ohlsson. A source for analgesia in newborn infants undergoing painful procedures (Cochrane Review). In: The Cochrane Library, Issue 3. Chichester: John Wiley, 2004.
22. Scottish Intercollegiate Guidelines Network (SIGN). *Safe sedation of children undergoing diagnostic and therapeutic procedures*. Guideline Number 58. Revised Edition, 2004.
23. Cote CJ. Effective and safe sedation for infants and toddlers undergoing procedures. In: David T. (ed) *Recent Advances in Paediatrics*, Vol. 21. London: The Royal Society of Medicine, 2004; 173–198.
24. Elliott CH, Olson RA. The management of children's distress in response to painful medical treatment for burn injuries. *Behav Ther Res* 1983; **21**: 675–683.
25. Jay SM, Elliott CH, Ozolins M, Olson RA, Pruitt SD. Behavioral management of children's distress during painful medical procedures. *Behav Ther Res* 1985; **23**: 513–520.

26. Duff AJA. Incorporating psychological approaches into routine paediatric venepuncture. *Arch Dis Child* 2003; **88**: 931–937.
27. Powers SW. Empirically supported treatments in pediatric psychology: procedure-related pain. *J Pediatr Psychol* 1999; **24**: 131–145.
28. Duff AJA, Ball R, Blyth H, Brownlee KG, Wolfe SP. *'Betterland'; an interactive CD-ROM guide for children with cystic fibrosis.* Welwyn Garden City: Roche Pharmaceuticals, 2004.
29. Jay SM, Elliott CH, Katz E, Siegel SE. Cognitive–behavioral and pharmacological interventions for children's distress during painful medical procedures. *J Consult Clin Psychol* 1987; **55**: 860–865.
30. Jay SM, Elliott CH, Woody PD *et al*. An investigation of cognitive–behavior therapy combined with oral valium for children undergoing medical procedures. *Health Psychol* 1991; **10**: 317–322.
31. Kazak A, Penati B, Boyer BA *et al*. A randomized controlled prospective outcome study of a psychological and pharmacological intervention protocol for procedural distress in pediatric leukemia. *J Pediatr Psychol* 1996; **21**: 615–631.
32. Willock J, Richardson J, Brazier A, Powell C, Mitchell E. Peripheral venepuncture in infants and children. *Nurs Standard* 2004; **18**: 43–50.
33. Royal Liverpool Children's NHS Trust. Policy Number RM 27. 2004.
34. Sullivan C, Schneider PE, Musselman RJ, Dummett Jr CO, Gardiner D. The effect of virtual reality during dental treatment on child anxiety and behavior. *ASDC J Dent Child* 2000; **67**: 193–196.
35. Hoffman HG, Doctor JN, Patterson DR, Carrougher GJ, Furness III TA. Virtual reality as an adjunctive pain control during burn wound care in adolescent patients. *Pain* 2000; **85**: 305–309.
36. Chen E, Zeltzer LK, Craske MG, Katz ER. Alteration of memory in the reduction of children's distress during repeated aversive medical procedures. *J Consult Clin Psychol* 1999; **67**: 481–490.
37. Lohr JM, Tolin DF, Kleinknecht RA. Eye movement desensitisation: two case studies. *J Behav Ther Exp Psychiatry* 1995; **26**: 141–151.
38. Ong EL, Lim NL, Koay CK. Towards a pain-free venepuncture. *Anaesthesia* 2000; **55**: 260–262.
39. Lysakowski C, Dumont L, Tramer MR, Tassonyi E. A needle-free jet-injection system with lidocaine for peripheral intravenous cannula insertion: a randomised controlled trial with cost-effectiveness analysis. *Anesth Analg* 2003; **96**: 215–219.
40. Stanley TH. Anesthetic techniques; a look into the future. Annual Refresher Course Lectures, 9–13 October 1999. American Society of Anesthesiologists.

Mary S. Fewtrell

12

Bone densitometry using dual X-ray absorptiometry (DXA)

Osteoporosis is a major and increasing cause of morbidity and mortality in industrialised countries, and is set to become so world-wide over the next 50 years. An individual's bone mass later in life is thought to be determined by the peak bone mass attained at skeletal maturity and by the subsequent rate of bone loss. Historically, strategies to prevent osteoporosis concentrated on reducing bone loss, particularly post-menopausally in women. However, over the past decade it has become clear that events operating during fetal life, infancy and childhood may affect peak bone mass and, therefore, potentially influence the development of osteoporosis.[1] Both nutritional factors and exercise are recognised as influential for normal skeletal development.

The appreciation that infancy and childhood are important periods of life for bone development has led to a need for suitable methods for monitoring bone health, both for research purposes and for clinical monitoring of individuals, and hence to an increasing use of bone densitometry (and related techniques) in children.

Bone densitometry was developed for use in adults to diagnose and monitor the course of osteoporosis, mainly in post-menopausal women. The most commonly used densitometric technique – dual X-ray absorptiometry (DXA) – was developed in the late 1980s and is now widely available. Other methods include axial and peripheral quantitative computed tomography (QCT), which can provide a three-dimensional assessment of the structural and geometric properties of the skeleton, plus a variety of methods using ultrasound to measure the speed and attenuation of

Mary S. Fewtrell BM BCh MD FRCPCH DCH
Honorary Senior Lecturer, MRC Childhood Nutrition Research Centre, Institute of Child Health, London & Great Ormond Street Hospital NHS Trust, 30 Guilford Street, London WC1N 1EH, UK
E-mail: m.fewtrell@ich.ucl.ac.uk

Abbreviations: CV, coefficients of variation; BMD, bone mineral density; aBMD, areal bone mineral density; BMC, bone mineral content; BA, bone area; BMAD, bone mineral apparent density; BMI, body mass index; BUA, broadband ultrasound attenuation; DXA, dual X-ray absorptiometry; ISCD, international consensus group; QCT, quantitative computed tomography; pQCT, peripheral quantitative computed tomography; QUS, quantitative ultrasound; SOS, speed of sound

sound through appendicular bone. Using these different techniques, measurements can be made of the whole body as well as regions such as the lumbar spine, hip and distal radius.

Areal measurements of bone mass – areal bone mineral density (areal BMD or aBMD) – made using DXA in untreated adults have been shown to predict a useful clinical outcome, namely fracture risk.[2] Indeed, World Health Organization (WHO) criteria for diagnosing osteoporosis in adults are based on DXA BMD measurements. Thus a T-score (defined as the standard deviation [SD] score of the observed BMD compared with that of a normal young adult) of ≤ 1 SD indicates osteopenia, whilst a score ≤ 2.5 SD defines osteoporosis.[3] The situation in children is very different. T-scores are meaningless, as they are the equivalent of comparing a child's height to that of an adult. Moreover, in children and younger adults, bone densitometry measurements have yet to be related to clinical outcome, and no fracture threshold has been defined. The use of these measurements, therefore, requires special care and consideration.

DXA BMD measurements are two-dimensional; they provide information about both bone size and bone density and are, therefore, highly related to body size. Children may have low bone mineral content (BMC) or areal BMD either because they have smaller bones and/or because they have less mineral than expected for the size of their bones (that is, genuinely reduced bone density). Current consensus is that it is worth distinguishing between these two factors, in terms of the underlying pathology and need for treatment.[4] Notwithstanding the above issues, when used appropriately, bone densitometry can be a useful tool in children. Its use falls into two categories:

RESEARCH

In this situation, bone densitometry is typically used to measure the effects of dietary or exercise interventions, often comparing randomised groups. There are fewer problems relating to the need to present the results for an individual in a clinically useful form. However, it is important to be able to interpret changes in bone density independent of those due to growth.

CLINICAL

In the clinical situation, patients are generally scanned either because they are thought to be at risk of low bone density because of their underlying disease or treatment, or to monitor the effects of treatment. One of the major problems with bone densitometry in individual patients is that of presenting results in a clinically useful form, given the factors discussed above. These issues are discussed further below.

This introduction has attempted to clarify why and how bone densitometry is currently being used in children, and some of the problems associated with such measurements. The remainder of this review will discuss:

1. How DXA works
2. Advantages of DXA in children
3. Limitations of DXA in children
   - Problems during data acquisition
   - Interpretation of results
   - Reference data

4. How DXA should be used in children
5. DXA in young adults
6. Other techniques for assessing bone mass or structure in children

HOW DXA WORKS

DXA determines the amount of mineral in a given region by the differential absorption of X-rays of two different energies – high and low. Low-energy photons are attenuated by soft tissue, whilst high-energy photons are attenuated by both bone and soft tissue; the amount of bone present can be quantified by subtracting one from the other. Using the same differential absorption, DXA can also take account of the depth and composition of adjacent soft tissue and generate measurements of fat and lean mass; this 'body composition' software is available on most machines with a whole body scan option. Using DXA, measurements can be made of the whole body as well as regions such as the lumbar spine, hip and distal radius. The choice of site may be important due to differences in the proportions of trabecular and cortical bone. Some conditions, such as steroid-induced bone loss, affect predominantly trabecular bone,[5] and may, therefore, be detected first at the lumbar spine. Others diseases, such as growth hormone deficiency, seem to cause greater deficits in cortical bone and may best be detected by scanning the whole body or distal radius.

Three companies currently manufacture DXA machines (GE Lunar, Hologic and Norland; the latter being a relatively smaller provider of machines). Each company produces more than one model. From the practical point of view, it is important to determine whether a machine is pencil-beam or fan-beam. Pencil-beam machines acquire data using a small-angle beam of X-rays that moves across the part being scanned in a recti-linear fashion. Fan-beam machines acquire data using a wider-angle beam. As a result, fan-beam machines have significantly lower scan times but the radiation doses are greater; obviously an important issue in children, particularly when collecting reference data from healthy individuals (Table 1). In addition, the use of a wide-angle beam introduces problems with magnification (see below). A

Table 1 Radiation doses from DXA compared to other procedures/activities

	Effective dose (μsV)
Lumbar spine DXA	0.4–4
Whole body DXA	0.02–5
Peripheral quantitative computed tomography	0.43 per slice
Quantitative computed tomography (spine)	55*
Hand X-ray	0.17
Chest X-ray	12–20
Lateral lumbar spine X-ray	700
Daily background radiation	6–20 (depending on location)
Return transatlantic flight	80

DXA values are the range for different machines
*Including lateral scan

recent addition to the GE Lunar family, the Prodigy, uses a combination of a narrow-angle fan beam with recti-linear scanning to give fast scan times with low radiation doses.

DXA has good precision, with reported coefficients of variation (CV) between 1% and 3% in adults. As investigators are generally reluctant to perform repeat measurements in children, specific coefficients of variation values for children are less clear. It is important to consider precision when interpreting apparent changes seen in longitudinal measurements.

ADVANTAGES OF DXA IN CHILDREN

DXA has a number of general advantages and also some that are particularly important for its use in children. Although the older pencil-beam machines took a considerable amount of time (up to 15 min) per scan, newer models are significantly faster, and it is possible to obtain scans of the lumbar spine in 2–3 min. This means that spine scans can be obtained in non-sedated children as young as 2.5–3 years.

Although DXA involves radiation, the exposure per scan (depending on machine and site) is generally in the range 0.4–5.4 µsV that is below a day's background radiation in the UK. This is obviously extremely important in children, both for clinical purposes, and when considering its use in healthy children to collect reference data.

LIMITATIONS OF DXA IN CHILDREN

PROBLEMS DURING DATA ACQUISITION

Different DXA machines give different results for a number of reasons relating to both the hardware and software used.

Machine calibration

GE Lunar machines consistently give BMD values around 16% higher than Hologic machines, partly because the former are calibrated to ashed bone, whilst Hologic machines are calibrated to hydroxyapatite. This can cause problems when children are scanned using different machines on different occasions, or in research when groups of subjects are scanned in centres with different machines. These problems can be to some degree circumvented by applying 'correction factors' to standardise measurements, although these have generally been derived in adults and not children.

Edge detection

DXA machines use algorithms to detect the edge of the bone being measured. These algorithms vary between machines, and, being designed for use in adults, may result in an inability to detect the bone edge in individuals with low bone density. Some machines have 'low density' or 'paediatric' software to overcome this problem, but it is important to appreciate that results obtained using these options cannot be directly compared to results obtained from standard or 'adult' software. Many machines will, by default, choose what they consider to be the most appropriate software based on the age or weight and height of the subject, although this can generally be over-ridden by the operator. The use of different software options even on the same machine can present problems when scanning an individual longitudinally where they cross from 'low' to 'normal' or from 'paediatric' to 'adult' software, or when scanning groups of subjects covering more than one software range. In this situation, it may be worth electing to use one software version consistently even though it may not be the one selected by the machine in all cases. However, care must be taken to ensure that this does not result in insufficient photons being available for analysis in some patients, for example, where a large individual is scanned using 'low density' software.

Magnification

This is a problem with fan-beam machines, because of differences in the distance between the bone and the X-ray source depending on the 'thickness' of the child. As the machines are designed for adult use, they are programmed to give 'correct' results at the distance expected in an average sized adult. However, the projected bone area and hence bone mineral content will vary in smaller (thinner) or larger (thicker) individuals, depending on where the bone is in relation to the X-ray source. Theoretically, magnification results in smaller errors in BMD (because errors in both bone mineral content and projected area should to some degree cancel each other out), but it makes interpretation of either bone mineral content or bone area measurements alone more difficult – this may be particularly relevant in children.

Effect of overlying tissue depth and composition

In vitro studies using bone phantoms with different overlying depths of fat, water and air demonstrate that both the thickness and composition of tissue surrounding a bone have an effect on measured BMD.[6] Unfortunately, these effects are generally not linear across the relevant range of tissue thickness, nor are they consistent between machines. Such effects may be relevant when patients are scanned longitudinally and have changes in body weight, because apparent changes in BMD may partly reflect alterations in body composition.[7,8]

REFERENCE DATA

Interpretation of DXA, particularly in a clinical context, relies on comparison with reference data. This is not such a problem in adult populations, for whom large data bases are generally available, but is a major issue in children. Most machines now incorporate a paediatric reference database, although the source is not always clear, and the numbers and ages of the children are generally not included. Machine reference databases typically provide bone mineral content or BMD for age, generally with separate reference data for boys and girls and sometimes for ethnic group, and a Z-score is generated. The use of sex-specific reference data is particularly important, as Leonard *et al.*[9] found that the use of sex-nonspecific reference data resulted in an overdiagnosis of osteopenia in boys. Weights and heights are generally not available for machine reference databases; this may be relevant when attempting to evaluate the effects of body size (see below).

The appreciation of the need for good quality, well documented reference databases has led paediatric investigators to collect their own reference data.

For example, in the UK, several groups are currently pooling data collected in healthy children, including anthropometry and ethnic group; the database will include data from > 1500 UK children. In the US, the National Institutes of Health are currently funding a national initiative for the collection of reference data, aiming to recruit 900 children. These databases should eventually be made generally available to interested parties.

INTERPRETATION OF DXA SCANS IN CHILDREN

For practical purposes, the information obtained from a DXA scan performed for clinical purposes should provide information about the likely existence and extent of bone disease and/or the risk of fracture. Alternatively, the scan may be used to provide information on the change in bone mass in response to disease or treatment. The former objective is currently difficult, because the predictive value of DXA measurements for clinical outcome has not been determined in children.

DXA machines measure bone mineral content (BMC) and bone area (BA) then calculate so-called bone mineral density (BMD) as BMC/BA. BMD is, therefore, not a true density, but a ratio of the amount of bone and the area scanned; it is a two-dimensional measurement that is affected by the subject's size. BMD will tend to underestimate true (volumetric) bone density in small subjects and over-estimate it in larger subjects. Most bone densitometers report BMD as a Z-score, related to an age-matched (and sometimes gender or ethnic-group matched) population.

Although the problem of size effects in bone densitometry is now widely appreciated, there is still no consensus on the most appropriate way to correct results for size, and express them. A number of different approaches have been suggested:

1. The use of calculated 'volumetric' bone density – termed bone mineral apparent density (BMAD), in which bone mineral content is adjusted for calculated bone volume rather than bone area. This approach can be used for spine and hip.[10,11]

2. A modification of the previous technique in which bone volume is additionally adjusted for height to correct for body size.[12]

3. The use of multiple regression analysis simultaneously to adjust bone mineral content for bone area, weight, height and other relevant factors such as age, pubertal status, calcium intake.[13,14]

4. A modification of the previous technique in which a staged approach is used, expressing height for age, bone area for height, and bone mineral content for bone area, to distinguish three potential situations in which reduced bone mass may occur; 'short' bones, 'narrow' bones and 'thin' bones.[15]

5. Calculation of the percentage predicted bone area, with subsequent calculation of the percentage predicted bone mineral content for measured bone area.[16]

6. A staged procedure incorporating lean mass, expressing bone mineral content for age, height for age, lean mass for height and finally bone mineral content divided by lean mass for height.[17]

7. Normalisation of bone mineral content or bone area for height[18] analogous to the use of weight adjusted for height in the body mass index (BMI).

All of the proposed methods recognise that bone mineral content or BMD measurements need to be interpreted in the context of the child's body size, pubertal stage and, to a lesser extent, age and ethnic group. The major problem with all methods is that it has not been possible to determine the predictive value of any of the proposed parameters for a meaningful outcome – thus effectively it is impossible to determine which method is 'best'.

A number of studies have demonstrated that using a size-corrected measure of bone mass significantly reduces the proportions of children diagnosed with a 'low' bone mass. For example, Gafni and Baron[19] reported that, of 34 children referred for possible inclusion in a childhood osteoporosis protocol based on the results of a DXA scan, 88% of scans had at least one error in interpretation. The most frequent error was the use of T-scores to diagnose osteoporosis, but in 15% of cases, errors resulted from a failure to consider the effect of short stature. When these errors were corrected, 53% of the children were considered to have normal BMD. Ahmed et al.[16] reported similar findings from a study using DXA in children with inflammatory bowel disease. Failure to account for reduced body size in the patient group led to a label of moderate or severe osteopenia in 65% of cases. This fell to 22% after adjustment for size. We recently examined four methods of size correction in groups of paediatric patients, and found that all size-corrected measures resulted in the classification of significantly fewer children as 'abnormal' when compared with bone mineral content or BMD; the four size-corrected measures in fact identified similar proportions (and the same individuals) as abnormal. Thus, in a practical clinical context, our data suggest that the precise method used for size correction may not be crucial. However, these data still fail to determine whether size-corrected methods give a more 'correct' verdict in terms of the prediction of true bone disease or fracture risk.

More recently, in an attempt to relate size-corrected measures to an outcome, Leonard et al.[18] used peripheral quantitative computed tomography measurements of the tibia (including a parameter of bone strength) as the 'gold standard'. They then tested in a group of 150 healthy children which size-corrected whole body DXA measurement best predicted the gold standard peripheral quantitative computed tomography outcomes. They found that bone area or bone mineral content normalised for height were the most predictive measures for tibial strength. Bone mineral content normalised for bone area or lean mass were poor predictors of bone strength in these analyses. The findings emphasise the importance of relating DXA measures to functional or clinical parameters rather than making assumptions about the most appropriate DXA parameters based on extrapolation of data from adult populations. It would be important, however, to determine whether bone mineral content or bone area normalised for height has the same predictive value in patient groups, where there may potentially be different relationships between bone mineral accretion and linear growth.

HOW SHOULD DXA BE USED IN CHILDREN?

RESEARCH

In the research situation, DXA may be used to measure the effects of dietary or exercise interventions, often comparing randomised groups. There are fewer

Bone densitometry using dual X-ray absorptiometry (DXA)

173

Table 2 Conditions in which children may be at increased risk of low bone density and osteoporotic fractures

Chronic inflammatory disease
Systemic long-term corticosteroids
Hypogonadism
Osteogenesis imperfecta
Idiopathic juvenile osteoporosis
Prolonged immobilisation
Apparent osteopenia on X-ray

problems relating to the need to present the results for an individual in a clinically useful form. However, it is important to be able to interpret changes in BMD independent of those due to growth; issues concerning size correction are, therefore, relevant although perhaps in a different way to those in individual patients. There may be problems if subjects are scanned on different machines or using different software as discussed above. When reporting results, it is important to specify the machine make, model and software version used, to enable comparison with other published data.

CLINICAL

In the clinical situation, patients are generally scanned either because they are thought to be at risk of low bone density because of their underlying disease or treatment, or to monitor the effects of treatment. Some conditions in which children are at increased risk are shown in Table 2. It has been suggested[4] that performance of a DXA scan should be considered if a child has one of these conditions in conjunction with one of the following symptoms: low trauma or recurrent fractures, back pain, spinal deformity or loss of height, change in mobility status (for example, difficulty walking), or malnutrition. This list is not exhaustive, but covers the conditions most commonly encountered. There are other, rarer conditions in which bone health may be altered and where assessment by DXA may be indicated (*e.g.* congenital neutropenia, certain

Table 3 Effects of body size on DXA measurements

	Patient 1	Patient 2
Patient	Male	Female
Weight (kg)	65	52
Weight SD score	0.29	−0.7
Height (cm)	161	163
Height SD score	−1.9	−0.08
BMD SD (Z) score	−2.3	−3.2
% expected bone area for age	74	104
% expected BM content for bone area	108	73
% expected BM apparent density for age	97	72
Interpretation	Short, small bones normal mineralisation	Normal size, low mineralisation

[BM = bone mineral]

inborn errors of metabolism, Ehlers Danlos syndrome, fibrous dysplasia, hypophosphatasia).

It is important to be aware that vertebral crush fractures may result in an artefactually high BMD value for the affected vertebra. This pitfall can be avoided by inspecting both the image and BMD for each vertebra scanned, and comparing vertebral size, rather than simply looking at the total lumbar spine BMD.

Since many children with chronic disease are small for their age, their BMD measurement will frequently appear to be low as well. This point is illustrated by the data in Table 3 from two children, both with chronic diseases. Both have low BMD Z-scores. However, patient 1 is short and has a low bone area for age, whilst patient 2 has normal weight, height and bone area for age. Two size-corrected measures of bone mass are shown. First, the percentage predicted BMC for measured BA, which is normal for patient 1 but low for patient 2. Second, the percentage predicted bone mineral apparent density (calculated volumetric bone density) which is also normal for patient 1 and low for patient 2. The conclusion is that patient 1 is short for his age and has small but normally mineralised bones, whilst patient 2, who is a normal size, has normal bone size but reduced mineral content. These results illustrate that the result of a DXA scan alone is insufficient for a diagnosis of abnormal bone mineralisation, and must be considered in conjunction with the clinical picture in order to avoid an inappropriate diagnosis.

Recently, an international committee of experts[20] made a statement regarding the diagnosis of osteoporosis in individuals less than 20 years of age. A modification of this has been adopted by the British Paediatric & Adolescent Bone Group (see Key Points).

At present, given the limitations discussed, a child may most appropriately act as his or her own control, with serial scans to monitor progress. Scan intervals of less than 6 months should only be considered in special situations such as monitoring the response to a pharmacological intervention, and for most patients annual scans should suffice. This approach will mean that the clinical and prognostic value of DXA should become apparent over the next few years, putting us in a better position to define the groups of children who most benefit from the investigation as well as to improve the prognostic value of a single measurement. It will also allow us to establish whether low BMD measurements that are considered to be a reflection of small body size have consequences for later bone health.

DXA SCANS IN YOUNG ADULTS

Although this article is primarily concerned with DXA in children, it is relevant to consider results obtained in young adults, particularly since many machines display T-scores together with WHO criteria for osteoporosis once subjects reach 20 years of age.

Some young adults have a low BMD for their age despite apparently normal weight and height, whilst others (for example, patients with certain chronic diseases and some individuals born preterm) remain small as adults, with a low BMD that is seemingly 'proportionate' for their reduced size. At present, it is not clear whether young adults with low BMD are at increased risk of developing osteoporosis later in life, and whether the risk might differ for those with low BMD proportionate to reduced body size compared to those with low BMD but normal size. Two studies in adult populations[21,22] found that, for individuals with the same low BMD, fracture risk was not affected by body size. This would suggest that young adults with low peak bone mass may well be at increased risk of future osteoporotic fractures, even if their low bone mass seems proportionate to their body size. Although other factors will undoubtedly be influential (for example, bone shape and geometry, plus bone turnover as well as environmental factors such as activity and diet), it may be unwise to assume that young adults with low peak bone mass will be protected from later fractures by 'proportionate' small body size.

Young adults with low bone mass measured by DXA present a problem in terms of management. A recent international consensus group (ISCD) considered these issues and made the following recommendations regarding the diagnosis of osteoporosis in young adults aged 20 years and over:[20]

1.   The WHO classification should not be applied to healthy premenopausal women, or men.

2.   Z-scores, not T-scores, should be used in this age group.

3.   The diagnosis of osteoporosis in premenopausal women or men under 50 years should not be made on the basis of densitometric criteria alone.

4.   Osteoporosis may be diagnosed if there is low BMD with secondary causes (*e.g.* glucocorticoid treatment, hypogonadism, hyperparathyroidism) or with risk factors for fracture.

In line with these recommendations, the most obvious option for young adults with low bone mass but no secondary causes or bone symptoms is to provide sensible advice regarding modifiable lifestyle factors such as calcium and vitamin D intake, and exercise. The more difficult issue to address is that of continued monitoring of bone mass. One option would be to recommend re-assessment in the event of future fragility fractures or bone pain, or possibly at the time of the menopause in women.

OTHER TECHNIQUES FOR ASSESSING BONE HEALTH IN CHILDREN

This review has concentrated on the use of DXA in children since this is by far the most commonly used method. However, other techniques have been used in the past, and/or are available today in a more limited capacity.

The earliest assessments of bone mass were made from conventional radiographs, using techniques such as the measurement of cortical thickness in appendicular bones, or radiographic densitometry where the optical density of the chosen bone was compared to that of a calibration aluminium step-wedge exposed simultaneously. All such methods had multiple problems, including the use of X-rays generated by a standard X-ray tube, the use of X-ray films to determine transmission rather than direct measurement of photons, and the inability to make adjustments for soft tissue. The net result was poor precision.

The development of absorptiometric techniques revolutionised the measurement of bone mass. These techniques are based on the exponential attenuation of photons as they pass through tissue. The earliest techniques used gamma-emitting sources to produce single or dual energy photon beams; such techniques were expensive since the gamma source had to be replaced at regular intervals, and they have now been superseded by X-ray based techniques such as DXA. Other X-ray based techniques such as quantitative computed tomography and peripheral quantitative computed tomography are also available but in a limited number of centres with a special interest in bone health and disease. Quantitative computed tomography methods allow a three-dimensional assessment of volumetric bone density, as well as the separation of cortical and trabecular bone compartments, measurement of cortical thickness and area, and parameters of bending strength in long-bones. The radiation exposure for quantitative computed tomography is generally considered too high for use in healthy children, but exposures for pquantitative computed tomography are acceptably low.

Quantitative ultrasound (QUS) has become more popular recently for assessing bone health, largely because it is portable, relatively cheap and involves no radiation. The technique measures the attenuation and speed of transmission of the ultrasound beam as it passes through bone and soft tissue, providing broadband ultrasound attenuation (BUA) and speed of sound (SOS) measurements. Most scanners to date measure the transmission of ultrasound through the bone (typically the calcaneus) using a transmitter placed on one side of the bone and a receiver on the other side. These machines have been designed primarily for use in adults. However, more recently developed machines using a single probe to measure the transmission of ultrasound longitudinally along a segment of bone (radius, tibia or phalanges) are suitable for use in small children and even neonates.

Ultrasound measurements are thought to reflect not only the density of the bone but also bone 'quality' or strength. In adult populations, broadband ultrasound attenuation and speed of sound measurements are predictive of fracture risk.[23,24] Studies in children have demonstrated differences in ultrasound measurements between patient groups and controls.[25,26] However, the predictive value of ultrasound measurements for fracture risk has not been determined in children and, therefore, the same limitations apply as already discussed for DXA. Ultrasound measurements are related to bone and body size; this is said to be less of a problem with machines measuring longitudinal transmission, although this is by no means proven. The extent to which DXA and ultrasound measurements are interchangeable (or provide the same information) is unclear and studies are currently underway to address this issue in different groups of children.

Key points for clinical practice

- The value of BMD measured by DXA for predicting fracture risk in children is not clearly determined.

- The WHO (T-score) classification of osteoporosis should not be applied in this age group

- T-scores should not be used in children: Z-scores (that is, age-matched)should be used instead.

(continued on next page)

(continued from previous page)

- T-scores should not appear in reports (this function should be switched off when the machine is used to scan children).

- The diagnosis of osteoporosis in children should not be based on densitometric criteria alone. Terms such as 'low bone density for age' may be used if the Z-score is ≤ 2.

- Z-scores must be interpreted in the light of the best available paediatric databases of age-matched controls. The reference database should be cited in the report.

- There is no consensus on standards for adjusting BMD or bone mineral content (BMC) for factors such as size, pubertal stage, skeletal maturity or body composition. If such adjustments are used, they should be clearly stated in the report.

- Serial BMD studies should be done on the same machine ideally using the same scanning mode, software and analysis, although changes may be required with growth.

- Any deviation from adult acquisition protocols – for example, the use of low density or paediatric software, or manual adjustment of regions of interest – should be stated in the report.

- It is recommended that DXA scans for 'clinical' reasons should not be performed outside centres with a clinical team with a specific interest and expertise in bone densitometry in children.

References

1. Javaid MK, Cooper C. Prenatal and childhood influences on osteoporosis. Best Practice Res Endocrinol Metab 2002; **16**: 349–367.
2. Cummings SR, Marcus R, Palermo L, Ensrud KE, Genant HK. Does estimated volumetric bone density of the femoral neck improve the prediction of hip fracture? A prospective study of the Osteoporotic Fracture Research Group. J Bone Miner Res 1994; **9**: 1429–1432.
3. WHO. Assessment of fracture risk and its application to screening for postmenopausal osteoporosis: report of a WHO study group. WHO Technical Report Series 843. Geneva: WHO, 1994.
4. Fewtrell MS and British Paediatric & Adolescent Bone Group. Bone densitometry in children assessed by dual x ray absorptiometry: uses and pitfalls. Arch Dis Child 2003; **88**: 795–798.
5. Bianchi ML. Glucocorticoids and bone: some general remarks and some special observations in pediatric patients. Calcif Tissue Int 2002; **70**: 384–390.
6. Laskey MA, Prentice A. Comparison of adult and paediatric spine and whole body software for the Lunar dual energy X-ray absorptiometer. Br J Radiol 1999; **72**: 967–976.
7. Bolotin HH. A new perspective on the causal influence of soft tissue composition on DXA-measured in vivo bone mineral density. J Bone Miner Res 1998; **13**: 1739–1746.
8. Tothill P, Laskey MA, Orphanidou CI, van Wijk M. Anomalies in dual energy X-ray absorptiometry measurements of total-body bone mineral during weight change using Lunar, Hologic and Norland instruments. Br J Radiol 1999; **72**: 661–669.
9. Leonard MB, Propert KJ, Zemel BS, Stallings VA, Feldman HI. Discrepancies in pediatric bone mineral density reference data: potential for misdiagnosis of osteopenia. J Pediatr 1999; **135**: 182–188.

10. Carter DR, Bouxsein ML, Marcus R. New approaches for interpreting projected bone densitometry data. *J Bone Miner Res* 1992; **7**: 137–145.
11. Kroger H, Kotaniemi A, Vainio P, Alhava E. Bone densitometry of the spine and femur in children by dual-energy X-ray absorptiometry. *Bone Miner* 1992; **17**: 75–85.
12. Smith CM, Coombs RC, Gibson AT, Eastell R. Approaches to adjusting bone mineral content for bone size in children. *Calcif Tissue Int* 2002; **70**: 370(A).
13. Prentice A, Parsons TJ, Cole TJ. Uncritical use of bone mineral density in absorptiometry may lead to size-related artefacts in the identification of bone mineral determinants. *Am J Clin Nutr* 1995; **60**: 837–842.
14. Warner JT, Cowan FJ, Dunstan FD, Evans WD, Webb DK, Gregory JW. Measured and predicted bone mineral content in healthy boys and girls aged 6–18 years: adjustment for body size and puberty. *Acta Paediatr* 1998; **87**: 244–249.
15. Molgaard C, Thomsen GL, Prentice A, Cole TJ, Michaelsen KF. Whole body bone mineral content in healthy children and adolescents. *Arch Dis Child* 1997; **76**: 9–15.
16. Ahmed SF, Horrocks IA, Patterson T *et al*. Bone mineral assessment by dual X-ray absorptiometry in children with inflammatory bowel disease: evaluation by age or bone area. *J Pediatr Gastroenterol Nutr* 2004; **38**: 276–281.
17. Hogler W, Briody J, Woodhead HJ, Chan A, Cowell CT. Importance of lean mass in the interpretation of total body densitometry in children and adolescents. *J Pediatr* 2003; **143**: 81–88.
18. Leonard MB, Shults J, Elliott DM, Stallings VA, Zemel BS. Interpretation of whole body dual X-ray absorptiometry measures in children: comparison with peripheral quantitative computed tomography. *Bone* 2004; **34**: 1044–1052.
19. Gafni RI, Baron J. Overdiagnosis of osteoporosis in children due to misinterpretation of dual-energy X-ray absorptiometry. *J Pediatr* 2004; **144**: 253–257.
20. The Writing Group for the ISCD Position Development Conference. Diagnosis of osteoporosis in men, premenopausal women and children. *J Clin Densitom* 2004; **7**: 17–26.
21. Albrand G, Munoz F, Sornay-Rendu E, DuBoeuf F, Delmas PD. Independent predictors of all osteoporosis-related fractures in healthy postmenopausal women: The OFELY Study. *Bone* 2003; **32**: 78–85.
22. Margolis KL, Ensrud KE, Schreiner PJ, Tabor HK. Body size and risk for clinical fractures in older women. *Ann Intern Med* 2000; **133**: 123–127.
23. Khaw KT, Reeve J, Luben R *et al*. Prediction of total and hip fracture risk in men and women by quantitative ultrasound of the calcaneus: EPIC-Norfolk prospective population study. *Lancet* 2004; **363**: 197–202.
24. Stewert A, Togerson DJ, Reid DM. Prediction of fractures in perimenopausal women: a comparison of dual energy X-ray absorptiometry and broadband ultrasound attenuation. *Ann Rheum Dis* 1996; **55**: 140–142.
25. Damilakis J, Galanakis E, Mamoulakis D, Sbyrakis S, Gourtsoyianis N. Quantitative ultrasound measurements in children and adolescents with Type 1 diabetes. *Calcif Tissue Int* 2004; **74**: 424–8.
26. Hartman C, Brik R, Tamir A, Merrick J, Shamir R. Bone quantitative ultrasound and nutritional status in severely handicapped institutionalized children and adolescents. *Clin Nutr* 2004; **23**: 89–98.

Jamiu O. Busari

13

Speech and language delay in children

Delay in speech and language development is the most common developmental disorder in children aged 3–16 years. The prevalence figures for speech and language disorders as a whole, range from 1% to 32% in the normal population and is influenced by several factors that include the age of the child at presentation, inclusion criteria, and the sort of test method used in diagnosis.[1–3] From these figures, it is thought that about 6% of children may have speech and language difficulties,[4] and that the aetiology in a significant proportion of this group could be attributed to a primary cause. A high rate of co-morbidity (up to 50%) is also found to exist between psychiatric disorders such as autism and disorders of speech and language development.[5] However, despite the prevalence and reported risks of co-morbidity, about 60% of these cases tend to resolve spontaneously in children aged less than 3 years.[1]

In clinical practice, clinicians are often faced with the dilemma of what to do when children with (primary) delays in their speech or language development are presented to them. Usually, the question is whether further investigations should be conducted to identify the cause of the disorder or to do nothing and see how the situation evolves. This is because in many cases, a delay in speaking could either be a normal (and temporary) phase in the child's development or the initial symptom of a psychiatric, neurological, or behavioural problem.[6] Furthermore, children with speech and language disorders are at an increased risk of developing difficulties with reading and written language when they enter school.[7–9]

In this chapter, special attention is paid to the definition and classification of speech and language delay in children. The different domains and the process of language development in the normal child are discussed and

Jamiu O. Busari MB ChB MHPE MD PhD
Consultant Paediatrician & Educationalist, Chief-attending, Department of Paediatrics, St Lucas Andreas Hospital, Jan Tooropstraat 164, 1006 AE Amsterdam, The Netherlands
E-mail: ojay33@hotmail.com

guidelines on how to identify and manage the child with a speech and language disorder are provided. The terms 'speech' and 'language' as well as 'delay' and 'disorder' are used interchangeably although they refer to the same concepts.

DEFINITIONS

Communication

Communication is the ability to receive, send, process and comprehend verbal as well as non-verbal concepts or graphic symbol systems. The normal development of communication requires the interaction between two systems, *i.e.* an intact mechanism and a favourable environment.[10] The components of an intact mechanism include: hearing sensitivity, perception, intelligence, structural integrity, motor skill, and emotional stability. A favourable environment on the other hand is a setting that provides a child with adequate language exposure and stimulation, reinforces the child's communicative attempts, and holds realistic expectations that are in tune with the child's developmental stage.

Language and speech

According to Berry,[11] language is a system of learned symbols that contain socially shared meanings and provides categories for classifying experiences. The production (and perception) of oral symbols is referred to as speech, while voice is the acoustic characteristics of both speech and non-speech sounds. The normal development of speech and/or language in children depends on the inter-relation among all of these different components. Any disturbance in the normal development, integration or inter-relation, of any (or all) of these components may result in a speech or language disorder. In the case of speech disorders, there is impairment in the articulation of speech sounds, fluency, and/or voice, while in language disorders the comprehension and/or use of spoken, written, and/or other symbol systems is impaired. Disorders of speech and/or language may involve the form (grammar, syntax, and morphology), content (vocabulary), and/or function (pragmatic use) of language.[10]

Speech and language delay/disorder

Providing a detailed and accurate description of disorders of speech and language development in children is complex. There are several definitions in the medical literature for speech and language development delay and most reflect the different methods and approaches that are used in the diagnosis of the impairment. Any definition of speech or language delay/disorder in children, however, should include one of two statements: (i) a delay in speech and/or language development in children compared with controls matched for age, sex, cultural background, and intelligence; or (ii) a discrepancy between a child's potential ability to speak and the performance that is actually observed.[6]

NORMAL LANGUAGE DEVELOPMENT

Language is a barometer of both cognitive and emotional development in children and includes both expressive and receptive functions. Receptive language (*i.e.* understanding) varies less in its rate of acquisition when compared to expressive language and is considered to be of more prognostic value than the latter. Although the timing of language acquisition and expression shows a great range of variation, the order of the language learning process in children is firm.[12] The variation in timing, however, may create difficulties for clinicians in discriminating normal (but delayed) language development in a child, from typical disorders of language or speech development. It might, therefore, be valuable for the clinician to have a prior understanding of normal language development in children before beginning to investigate a speech or language disorder in a child.

Domains of language development

The study of language is focused mainly on: (i) its sounds; (ii) organisation within and between words; (iii) the organisation of concepts; and (iv) its use. Most linguists refer to these domains as phonology, grammar, semantics, and pragmatics, which are relatively dissociable and governed by certain rules. As shown by the tight sequence in which the component elements of language emerge, they are strongly interdependent and constrain each other.[13] The development of the different domains of language is marked by a predictable and expected developmental course, which is associated with: (i) reception and expression; (ii) encoding and decoding; (iii) comprehension and production; and (iv) the underlying competencies and manifest performances.[2] To illustrate this process, a brief summary of the four domains of language is provided below.

Phonology
Phonology refers to the ability to produce and discriminate the specific sounds of a given language. Its unit is the phoneme, *e.g.* /p/ or /b/, characterised by their distinctive features. The /p/ and /b/ phonemes are distinguished by the 'voiced' quality of /b/, *i.e.* the vocal cord vibration that ensues after the initial sound versus the lack of vibration in /p/. Phonological receptivity to different languages is optimal at birth but starts to decline at about age 10 months. There is a general inability to acquire native phonology by pre-adolescence.[14]

Grammar
Grammar refers to the underlying rules that organise any specific language. In linguistics, it comprises the rules that govern the combination of words in a language, which the native speakers of the language recognise as acceptable. Grammar is composed of both **morphology** (*i.e.* within word structure) and **syntax** (*i.e.* between words structure). Morphology studies the smallest word unit that impacts on meaning (*i.e.* the morpheme). An illustration of morphology is the word *autos* which is constituted by the morpheme, *auto* (base morpheme) and –*s* (inflectional morpheme denoting plural). *Autism* on the other hand comprises of the base morpheme *auto* (denoting oneself) which is joined by a derivational morpheme –*ism* (denoting 'typical qualities').

Syntax refers to the set of rules that governs the types of words (*e.g.* subject, verb, object, adverb), their order (*e.g.* subject-verb-object-adverb in English, subject-object-adverb-verb in Dutch), the rigidity of the order (*e.g.* highly rigid English, flexible in Spanish), and the way to formulate a question or a negation (using auxiliary verbs or not), *etc.* Children start to learn grammar when they start to speak about objects, people and actions. Although the core grammatical rules seem to be the result of the interaction between universal grammar and the environmental language, more complex grammatical development, such as appreciation of the passive voice, appears to be highly correlated to the quality and quantity of input and interaction.[2]

Semantics

Semantics is the study of meaning and includes the study of vocabulary (lexicon). Lexical entries are organised in the mental dictionary according to well-defined rules, which allow the young child to acquire a peak average of 10 new words per day. By 24 months, the average child knows about 50–100 words. The exponential growth in vocabulary that ensues hereafter makes it difficult to determine accurately a child's vocabulary size, which is thought to be the best predictor of school success.[1] The acquisition of morphology also makes the possible combinations of words much larger. Environmental factors known to predict large vocabularies in children include reading and discussing children's stories, the quality of dinner table conversations, higher socio-economic status, being the first-born and the quantity and sophistication of mother's vocabulary.[15,16]

Pragmatics

Pragmatics refers to the ability of the child to use his or her language in interactions with others. It comprises a number of sub-domains that reflect communicative competence. These include, for example, the rules of conversation (*i.e.* turn-taking, topic maintenance, conversational repair), of politeness, of narrative and extended discourse and of the implementation of communicative intents. These features of pragmatics have distinct developmental trajectories and constitute the scaffolding for the emergence of lexicon, then grammar, and eventually narrative.[13,16,17]

Acquisition of language

The acquisition of language depends critically on environmental input and the key determinants include the amount and variety of speech that is directed towards the child, as well as the frequency with which adults ask questions and encourage verbalisation. Child abuse and neglect, for example, are correlated with delayed language development in children particularly in their ability to convey emotional states. Furthermore, class-related disparities in preschool language development and later school achievement have been associated with the striking differences in the parameters between upper- and lower-class parents.[15,16]

Many linguists believe that the basic mechanism for language learning is 'hard-wired' in the brain and that children do not simply imitate adults. Rather, they abstract the complex rules of grammar from the ambient language and generate implicit hypotheses.[18] The normal language learning process in children shows that they start babbling at 6–10 months, understand words by 8–10 months and, on average, most children speak their first words around their first birthday. In the second year, receptive language precedes expressive language. By 12–18 months, most children respond appropriately to several simple statements such as 'yes', 'bye-bye' and 'give me'. From the 15th month, the average child can point to major body parts and can use 4–6 words spontaneously and correctly. By age 18–24 months, labelling of objects co-incides with the advent of symbolic thought. Children may point at things with their index finger rather than their whole hand as though calling attention to objects not for the purpose of having them, but of finding out their names. The realisation that words can stand for things increases the child's vocabulary from 10–15 words at 18 months to 100 or more at 2 years. Children start to combine words to form sentences as soon as they have acquired a vocabulary of about 50 words, marking the beginning of grammar development. At this stage, toddlers understand two-step commands such as 'give me the spoon and then drink your milk'. The emergence of verbal language marks the end of the sensorimotor period as toddlers learn to use symbols to express ideas and solve problems. Between the ages of 2–5 years, language development tends to be rapid. Vocabulary increases from a 100 to more than 2000 words. Sentence structure advances from telegraphic phrases ('baby cry') to sentences incorporating all of the major grammatical components. As a rule of thumb, between 2 and 5 years of age, the number of words in a typical sentence equals the child's age, *i.e.* 2 words by age 2, 3 words by age 3, *etc.* By the age of 4 years, clear syntax is part of most children's speech.[18,19]

MANAGEMENT OF SPEECH AND LANGUAGE DELAY

Evaluation of speech and language impairment in children

Parents of children with symptoms of delayed speech and language development usually approach a clinician when the child is between 2 and 3 years of age. Their concerns that something may be wrong at such moments should be taken seriously as parents' observations of abnormal behaviour in children at this age are quite accurate.[20] In older children, however, preschool and school records may be the resources that clinicians may have to rely on in identifying any signs of delayed speech or language development.[5] At present, there is no known clear-cut approach in the medical literature on how to manage children with speech or language delay. This is because external factors such as the cause of the delay, the severity of presenting symptoms, availability of screening, and treatment facilities (may) vary enormously. Nevertheless, it is recommended that any evaluation of speech and language impairment in children should include: (i) determining whether there is an identifiable impairment in the child's communication; (ii) specifying the nature of the impairment, if any; and (iii) initiating an appropriate and timely intervention strategy (Box 1).

A guideline that may be helpful for clinicians in investigating and managing a child who is slow to speak is provided in this section. The

---

Box 1 Criteria for speech and language evaluation

- Concern by parent, teacher, professional or other care-giver about a child's speech or language
- Delay in a child's speech and language development
- Difficulty in sucking, chewing, swallowing, or excessive drooling
- Abnormal co-ordination of lips, tongue and jaw in a child
- No babbling by 9 months
- No first words by 15 months
- No consistent words by 18 months
- No word combinations or parents have difficulty understanding speech by 24 months
- Speech is difficult for others to understand at 36 months
- Dysfluencies (stutters) consist of more than tension-free whole word repetitions
- Frustration in child with communication difficulty
- Child avoids talking situations or is teased by peers for 'talking funny'
- Language is unusual or confused, or ideas are not expressed clearly
- Child cannot follow instructions without supplemental cues
- Loss or delay of developmental milestones
- Poor memory skills at 5–6 years

From Carter and Musher.[42]

---

components of the guideline are derived from the evidence in the medical literature and the outline, although empirical, is meant to serve as a pragmatic resource that can be used during an office consultation (see Fig. 1). The guideline's objective is to assist clinicians (and speech therapists) in effectively determining the sort, cause, and severity of speech and/language disorders in children, as well as choosing appropriate forms of intervention.

Box 2 Precursors of normal speech and language development in children

- Playing meaningfully with toys
- Interacting appropriately with others
- Demonstrating the ability to understand the world around him or her
- Imitating body gestures, sounds, syllables
- Adequately comprehending simple verbal instructions

From Carter and Musher.[42]

---

18. Needlam RD. Growth and development. In: Behrman RE, Kliegman RM, Jenson HB. (eds) *Nelson Textbook of Pediatrics,* 17th edn. Philadelphia, PA: Saunders, 2004; 44–53.

19. Crosley CJ. Speech and language disorders. In: Swaiman KF, Ashwai S. (eds) *Pediatric Neurology, Principles and Practice.* Minneapolis: Mosby, 1999, 568–575.

20. Wetherby AM, Allen L, Cleary J, Kublin K, Goldstein H. Validity and reliability of the communication and symbolic behaviour scales developmental profile with very young children. *J Speech Lang Hear Res* 2002; **45**: 1202–1218.

21. Shaywitz SE, Escobar MD, Shaywitz BA, Fletcher JM, Makuch R. Evidence that dyslexia may represent the lower tail of a normal distribution of reading ability. *N Engl J Med* 1992; **326**: 145–150.

22. Roberts JE, Rosenfeld RM, Zeisel SA. Otitis media and speech and language: a meta-analysis of prospective studies. *Pediatrics* 2004; **113**: 238–248.

23. Coplan J, Gleason JR. Quantifying language development from birth to three years using the early language milestone development scale. *Pediatrics* 1990; **86**: 963–971.

24. Cronin VS. The syntagmatic-paradigmatic shift and reading development. *J Child Lang* 2002; **29**: 189–204.

25. Tomblin JB. Perspectives on diagnosis. In: Tomblin JB, Morris LH, Spriestersbach DC. (eds) *Diagnosis in Speech-Language Pathology.* San Diego, CA: Singular Publishing, 2000; 3–33.

26. Tallal P, Miller S, Fitch RH. Neurobiological basis of speech: a case for the pre-eminence of temporal processing. *Ann NY Acad Sci* 1993; **682**: 27–47.

27. Semrud-Clikeman M. Evidence from imaging on the relationship between brain structure and developmental language disorders. *Semin Pediatr Neurol* 1997; **4**: 117–124.

28. Gauger LM, Lombardino LJ, Leonard CM. Brain morphology in children with specific language impairment. *J Speech Lang Hear Res* 1997; **40**: 1272–1284.

29. Gigler JW. Genetics in disorders of language. *Clin Commun Disord* 1992; **2**: 35–47.

30. Rice ML, Haney KR, Wexler K. Family histories of children with SLI who show extended optional infinitives. *J Speech Lang Hear Res* 1998; **41**: 419–432.

31. Tallal P, Ross R, Curtiss S. Familial aggregation in specific language impairment. *J Speech Hear Disord* 1989; **54**: 167–173.

32. Shriberg LD. Five subtypes of developmental phonological disorders. *Clin Commun Disord* 1994; **4**: 34–53.

33. Piven J, Palmer P, Jacobi D, Childress D, Arndt S. Broader autism phenotype: evidence from a family history study of multiple-incidence autism families. *Am J Psychiatry* 1997; **154**: 185–190.

34. Snow C. Beginning from baby talk: twenty years of research on input and interaction. In: Galloway C, Richards B. (eds) *Input and Interaction in Language Acquisition.* London: Cambridge University Press, 1994; 3–12.

35. Hoff-Gingsberg E. The relation of birth disorder and socio-economic status to children's language experience and language development. *Child Dev* 1991; **62**: 782–796.

36. Beals DE, De Temple JM, Dickinson DK. Talking and listening that support early literacy development of children from low-income families. In: Dickinson DK. (ed) *Bridges to Literacy: Children, Families, and Schools.* Cambridge: Blackwell, 1994; 19–40.

37. Lewis BA, Cox NJ, Byard PJ. Segregation analysis of speech and language disorders. *Behav Genet* 1993; **23**: 291–297.

38. Seymour HN, Bland L. A minority perspective in the diagnosis of child language disorders. *Clin Commun Disord* 1991; **1**: 39–50.

39. Hancock K, Craig A, McCready C *et al.* Two- to six-year controlled-trial stuttering outcomes for children and adolescents. *J Speech Lang Hear Res* 1998; **41**: 1242.

40. Gierut JA. Treatment efficacy: functional phonological disorders in children. *J Speech Lang Hear Res* 1998; **41**: S85.

41. Law J, Garrett Z, Nye C. Speech and language therapy interventions for children with primary speech and language delay or disorder (Cochrane Review). In: *The Cochrane Library*, Issue 1, 2004. Chichester, UK: John Wiley.

42. Carter J, Musher K. Evaluation and treatment of speech and language impairment in children, 2004, *UpToDate online* 12.2 <www.uptodate.com> accessed 30 June 2004.

Anthony W. Solomon   David C.W. Mabey

14

Trachoma

Trachoma causes blindness in poor people. It develops as a result of repeated ocular infection with *Chlamydia trachomatis*. Though the highest prevalence of infection occurs in childhood, in most trachoma-endemic communities, blinding complications are generally not seen until middle or old age. As a result, trachoma usually attracts the attention of ophthalmologists, infectious disease physicians and public health specialists, rather than paediatricians. It is important, though, that paediatricians are updated about trachoma, for three reasons. First, in areas of extremely intense transmission, where the prevalence of infection in young children approaches 100%, the blinding complications of trachoma are seen in paediatric patients. Second, in all endemic areas, the seeds of trachoma blindness are sown in childhood. Clinical recognition of active trachoma in the eyes of children attending medical clinics for other reasons should lead to assessment of the community and, if indicated, community-based trachoma control efforts. Such interventions may prevent blindness in hundreds or thousands of individuals. Third, trachoma has been targeted by the World Health Organization (WHO) for elimination as a cause of blindness by the year 2020. All medical professionals have an interest in disease control and elimination, and their support, directly or indirectly, will be critical to ensuring that this goal is achieved.

MICROBIOLOGY

The contagious nature of trachoma was recognised in Syria in the 13th century, but the causative agent was not visualised until Halberstaedter and von

Anthony W. Solomon MBBS PhD DTM&H
Lecturer in International Eye Health

David C.W. Mabey DM FRCP (for correspondence)
Professor, Clinical Research Unit, London School of Hygiene & Tropical Medicine, Keppel Street, London WC1E 7HT, UK
E-mail: david.mabey@lshtm.ac.uk

Prowazek found what they thought were protozoa inside infected conjunctival cells in 1907.[1] A further 50 years then passed before T'ang and colleagues completed the first successful isolation of the organism. Because it filtered through 400×10^{-9}-m diameter membrane pores, it was assumed to be a virus.[2] Subsequent research clarified details of its structure, chemical composition, metabolism and developmental cycle, and eventually *Chlamydia* was definitively re-classified as a genus of intracellular bacteria. Chlamydiae rely on host cells for survival and replication because they lack cytochromes and, therefore, can not synthesize their own ATP.

Based originally on binding affinity for monoclonal antibodies (and, more recently, on corresponding polymorphisms in genes coding for a major surface-exposed protein), *C. trachomatis* has been divided into a number of serovars. Serovars A, B, Ba and C preferentially infect epithelial cells of the conjunctiva, and are associated with trachoma, while serovars D to K, Da, Ia and Ja preferentially infect mucosal epithelium of the urogenital tract. The rare L1, L2, L2a and L3 serovars can invade lymphatic tissue, and are associated with lymphogranuloma venereum.

The first complete *C. trachomatis* genome sequence was published in 1998.[3] Recently, it has been established that ocular strains have a deletion or frame-shift mutation in a region encoding for enzymes important in tryptophan synthesis, while genital strains do not.[4] This finding is the first known point of biochemical difference between ocular and genital isolates of *C. trachomatis*.

CLINICAL AND PATHOLOGICAL FEATURES

Clinically and pathologically, the manifestations of trachoma are divided into acute (active) and chronic (late-stage). However, trachoma has a multi-cyclic course, requiring repeated *C. trachomatis* infections – each of which may be associated with an episode of active disease – for later development of the chronic sequelae.[5] It is, therefore, possible for acute and chronic signs to be present simultaneously in the same eye.

For several weeks after infection, the only visible clinical sign is conjunctival hyperaemia. Lymphoid follicles, the hallmark of active trachoma, then develop subjacent to the conjunctival epithelium. Macroscopically, these appear as creamy or grey masses with a diameter of 0.2–3.0 mm. Histologically, follicles are dense collections of inflammatory cells, including B- and T-lymphocytes, plasma cells, monocytes, and macrophages. Mature follicles have pale-staining germinal centres surrounded by a mantle of proliferating lymphocytes. The nucleus of a germinal centre contains metabolically active plasma cells. Both CD8+ and CD4+ T-lymphocytes are recruited as part of the inflammatory response to acute infection, with CD8+ T-cells predominating.[6] The conjunctival epithelium is generally hyperplastic, though thinning is observed over follicles. Infected cells contain inclusion bodies, which are membrane-bound cytoplasmic vacuoles in which chlamydiae grow and divide. Papillae (small elevations of the conjunctiva, each with a central vascular core) are also associated with active trachoma. The intensity of the papillary reaction indicates the severity of active inflammation: at its most intense, the conjunctiva becomes diffusely thickened, and the normal deep conjunctival vessels can no longer be visualised through the epithelial layer. In the peripheral cornea, sub-epithelial infiltration of fibrovascular tissue, known as pannus, may accompany active disease, and may persist long after the signs of conjunctival inflammation have disappeared. Most ocular *C. trachomatis* infections are asymptomatic. Some infected individuals report an irritable red eye with scanty discharge.

Resolution of follicles may be accompanied by scarring of the sub-epithelial conjunctiva. In conjunctival tissue with late-stage disease, there is a proliferation of fibroblasts, and deposition of vertically oriented, parallel collagen fibres in a layer adherent to the tarsal plate. This scar tissue replaces the normal thin, loose, vascular stroma,[7] and when profuse, becomes visible to the naked eye in the everted conjunctiva. Translucent depressions known as Herbert's pits may form following resolution of follicles at the sclero-corneal junction. Meibomian glands are infiltrated by lymphocytes, and are atrophic or deformed by scarring. The epithelium is also atrophic, with a reduction in the number of columnar epithelial cells. Goblet cells are absent.

Contraction of scars produced over many years may eventually cause the eyelid to invert, so that the lashes touch the globe. This condition, which is known as trichiasis, is intensely irritating, and impairs vision by provoking corneal oedema and blepharospasm. When the central lashes are affected, trichiasis abrades the cornea. Constant corneal trauma leads to its scarring and opacification; corneal blindness may be the result. Histologically, in the scarred cornea, there is degeneration and irregularity in the thickness of the epithelium, and disorganisation of the normal perpendicular orientation of the collagen lamellae in the stroma, sometimes with calcification. Capillaries or ghost vessels may be seen in the superficial and middle stromal layers.

IMMUNITY AND PATHOGENESIS

THE IMMUNE RESPONSE TO *C. TRACHOMATIS* INFECTION

The innate immune system responds to the presence of chlamydiae. There is an influx of neutrophils to the site of infection, and production of pro-inflammatory cytokines, including interleukin-1α , interleukin-1β, platelet-derived growth factor, and tumour necrosis factor-α, by infected epithelial cells and conjunctival macrophages. Unfortunately, inflammatory responses may be responsible for some of the tissue damage associated with infection, and may not necessarily clear the organism from the epithelium.

Strain-specific protective immunity against ocular (or genital) *C. trachomatis* infection seems to be induced by repeated infection. In trachoma-endemic communities, induction of anti-chlamydial immunity seems likely to underlie the observed decrease in the duration of both infection and disease with age, and the increase in intensity of inflammation in those shorter disease episodes of older people.[8] Precise mechanisms for the development of the adaptive immune response are unclear. Cytokines released as part of the innate response (which are predominantly of the Th-1 type) likely contribute to initiating adaptive immunity, and both cell-mediated and antibody-mediated systems seem to be recruited. Whilst antibodies probably make a modest contribution to protection against re-infection, in the mouse model they are not essential for it.[9] It is also possible that anti-chlamydial IgG in tears actually enhances the infectivity of *C. trachomatis* for human conjunctival epithelium.[10]

Cell-mediated immune mechanisms (the Th-1 response), and CD4[+] cells in particular, seem to be critical in clearing infection.[9,11] There is evidence that individuals who develop scarring do not have adequate anti-chlamydial Th-1 responses. In lymphocyte proliferation assays, peripheral blood mononuclear cells of individuals with conjunctival scarring have reduced responses to *C. trachomatis* antigens compared to matched control subjects, but equivalent responses to other antigens.[12] Class II major histocompatibility complex molecules (which present antigen to CD4[+] T-lymphocytes) are not found on conjunctival epithelial cells in most populations, but are found on conjunctival epithelial cells of patients with ocular *C. trachomatis* infections in trachoma-endemic communities.[13] In animal models, there is a marked increase in the number of CD4[+] cells in conjunctival tissue after experimental inoculation with this organism.[6]

VIRULENCE FACTORS OF *C. TRACHOMATIS*

Intracellular chlamydiae inhibit phagosome–lysosome fusion (by mechanisms that are yet to be defined). This allows the organism to survive and replicate within conjunctival epithelial cells. Eventually, host conjunctival tissues are damaged. Three putative *C. trachomatis*-derived pro-inflammatory factors, which may be involved in generating this damage, have been identified:

1. The chlamydial heat shock protein (hsp)-60 induces a delayed-type hypersensitivity response in the conjunctivae of previously sensitised experimental animals.[14] In humans, serum antibodies to this protein have been associated with scarring, though whether anti-hsp-60 itself contributes to immunopathology or is simply found more commonly in people with long standing infection is not known.[15]

2. Proteins homologous to the large cytotoxins A and B of *Clostridium difficile*[16] induce host cell rounding and cytoskeletal collapse – changes identical to those induced by clostridial cytotoxin B.

3. Chlamydial proteasome-like activity factor, or CPAF, may be involved in down-regulating expression of class II major histocompatibility complex molecules[17] by infected cells and may, therefore, help chlamydiae evade immune recognition.

There is little to suggest that there are major differences in inherent virulence between different ocular serovars of *C. trachomatis*.

PRESSURE OF INFECTION

A single episode of *C. trachomatis*-stimulated conjunctival inflammation resolves in weeks or a few months, even without treatment. Conjunctival scarring produced by a single infection is unlikely to produce trichiasis. In trachoma hyperendemic areas, however, recrudescence or re-infection occurs within weeks or months of resolution of the previous episode of active disease. The actual number, duration and intensity of infections required for the accumulation of pathologically significant scar in the human conjunctiva is not known.

GENETIC SUSCEPTIBILITY

Longitudinal studies suggest that some individuals are more likely than others to develop severe inflammatory changes in response to conjunctival *C. trachomatis* infection.[18] The duration of severe disease seems to be related to the ability of the host to clear infection.[19] Persistent severe disease is associated with later development of conjunctival scar.[20] These results suggest that variability in the host response to *C. trachomatis* infection in part determines an individual's risk for developing scarring complications and, therefore, possibly blindness from trachoma. Case-control studies in The Gambia have identified associations between conjunctival scarring and both class II major histocompatibility complex alleles[21] and polymorphisms in the tumour necrosis factor-α gene promoter.[22]

PATHOGENESIS OF CORNEAL OPACITY

Corneal damage by in-turned eyelashes is generally assumed to be the ultimate mechanism for blindness due to trachoma. Other features of the trachomatous eye probably also contribute. In particular, scarring of forniceal mucous, lacrimal and Meibomian glands (which reduces their secretory output and therefore dries the eye), and a reduction in the concentrations of lysozyme and lactoferrin in tear fluid, predispose the cornea to secondary bacterial and fungal infections, which generate an additional burden of corneal scar.

DIAGNOSIS

Examination for the clinical signs of trachoma involves careful inspection for in-turned lashes, pannus, Herbert's pits and corneal opacities, then gentle eversion of the upper lid and inspection of the tarsal conjunctiva. To evert the lid, the patient is instructed to look down without closing their eyes. The examiner uses a thumb and first or second finger to gently pull downwards on the patient's lashes, places the little finger of his or her other hand (or a small, blunt, smooth tool, such as a matchstick) at the upper edge of the tarsal plate, and folds the lid backwards over that fixed point. Eversion is maintained by holding the patient's lashes against their orbital margin with the thumb. If the patient is a child, an assistant is usually required. Binocular magnifying loupes (2.5×) are used to examine for follicles and papillary inflammation. The examination should be conducted in sunlight or with a torch (sunlight is preferable). Follicles smaller than 0.5 mm in diameter and those at the medial or lateral canthus are ignored, since these may be normal, particularly in children.

Most trachoma surveys and national trachoma programmes use the WHO's simplified grading system[23] to assess communities and to monitor the success of control efforts. This system was not intended for use in the assessment of individual patients. For that purpose, a history of living in a trachoma-endemic area and the full clinical picture should be considered. The WHO simplified system is presented here, however, to help readers understand the literature on trachoma.

The simplified system requires the examiner to assess an individual for the presence or absence of each of five signs (Fig. 1):

(A) Normal conjunctiva, showing area to be examined

(B) TF

(C) TI (and TF)

(D) TS

(E) TT

(F) CO

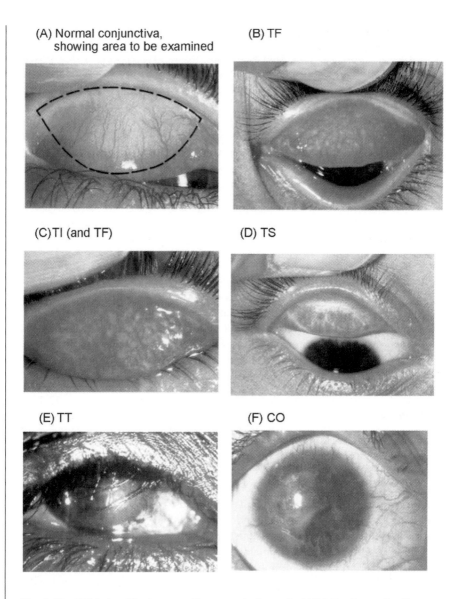

Fig. 1 The WHO simplified system. Photographs from the WHO Trachoma Grading Card (© World Health Organization, reproduced with permission).

TF **Trachomatous inflammation – follicular**: the presence of five or more follicles at least 0.5 mm in diameter, in the central part of the upper tarsal conjunctiva.

TI **Trachomatous inflammation – intense**: pronounced inflammatory thickening of the upper tarsal conjunctiva obscuring more than half the normal deep tarsal vessels.

TS **Trachomatous conjunctival scarring**: the presence of easily visible scars in the tarsal conjunctiva.

TT **Trachomatous trichiasis**: at least one eyelash rubs on the eyeball, or evidence of recent removal of in-turned eyelashes.

CO **Corneal opacity**: easily visible corneal opacity over the pupil, so dense that at least part of the pupil margin is blurred when viewed through the opacity

TF is a manifestation of moderately severe active disease, while TI is a manifestation of severe active disease. In the simplified system, the presence of TF and/or TI in an eye is taken to indicate 'active trachoma'.

LABORATORY TESTS FOR *C. TRACHOMATIS*

Trachoma is a disease of poor communities. Laboratory assays are expensive. As a result, trachoma is a diagnosis that is almost always made on clinical grounds alone. However, not everyone with an ocular *C. trachomatis* infection has clinical signs of active trachoma, and – particularly after antibiotic treatment – not everyone with clinical signs has an ocular *C. trachomatis* infection. This has implications for determining which individuals and communities need trachoma control interventions, and for the criteria that will be used to certify elimination of trachoma. These issues are presently the subject of research.

If tests for infection are to be used to guide trachoma control efforts, which assay or assays should be used? Available tests include microscopic examination of stained conjunctival scrapings for inclusion bodies, culture, immunofluorescence, EIA, and nucleic acid amplification tests such as PCR. Though the nucleic acid amplification tests are technically complex and very expensive, they are thought to be the most sensitive for detecting *C. trachomatis* infection. They are also highly specific. These tests are, therefore, valuable in trachoma research studies, and are likely to play a role in helping to develop guidelines for certification of trachoma elimination.

Tissue culture is known to be imperfectly sensitive, and is difficult, expensive and time-consuming to perform. However, it is nearly 100% specific, and a positive test demonstrates that viable *C. trachomatis* (not just nucleic acid) was present in the sample. Additionally, in specialised laboratories, culture may be used to determine the antimicrobial susceptibilities of *C. trachomatis* isolates. The need to undertake surveillance for the emergence of antimicrobial resistance will be mentioned below.

EPIDEMIOLOGY

IMPORTANCE AS A CAUSE OF BLINDNESS

The most recent published estimates of the global prevalence and causes of blindness were based on vastly incomplete data, and are now over a decade old. They suggest that there were about 5.9 million people blind due to trachoma in 1990, making it the second most common cause of blindness after cataract.[24] Further work to quantify the global public health problem posed by trachoma is needed urgently to aid planning for disease elimination. There are probably 600 million people living in trachoma-endemic areas in Africa, the Middle East, Central and South America, Asia, Australia, and the Pacific Islands.

RISK FACTORS FOR DISEASE AND INFECTION

Trachoma is strongly associated with poverty. Affected communities tend to live in remote areas and have grossly inadequate access to water, sanitation and health care.

The prevalence of clinical signs of active disease rises to a peak in children in the immediate pre-school years. Thereafter, prevalence of active disease declines with age. The prevalence of ocular *C. trachomatis* infection is also highest in children. In endemic communities, individuals under 10 years of age probably harbour the bulk of the reservoir of ocular *C. trachomatis*.[25]

Scarring complications and blindness from trachoma are seen more commonly with increasing age. Perhaps because of their greater involvement in the care of children, the risk of every sign of trachoma is greater in women than in men.

MECHANISMS OF TRANSMISSION

The actual mechanisms of transmission of ocular *C. trachomatis* infection are unproven. Eye-seeking flies (particularly the bazaar fly, *Musca sorbens*[26]), fingers, and shared cloths, towels and bedding are probably involved. Since *C. trachomatis* is found in the nasopharynx and external nasal secretions of people living in trachoma-endemic communities, it seems likely that droplet transmission may also play a role.

TREATMENT AND PREVENTION

The only effective treatment for corneal blindness is keratoplasty, which generally involves the placement of a full-thickness corneal graft. In the trachomatous eye, reduced tear secretion, corneal vascularisation and distortion of the lid all tend to worsen graft prognosis. In any case, logistical and financial constraints mean that trachoma-endemic countries are generally unable to support corneal grafting programmes.

The focus of trachoma control programmes, therefore, needs to be preventative. Unfortunately, a vaccine capable of invoking useful immunity to ocular chlamydial infection is unlikely to become available within the next decade. Current strategies for the management and control of trachoma are aimed at interrupting the pathogenic cascade that leads to blindness: reduction in transmission of infection from person-to-person through fly control and the removal of infected ocular secretions from children's faces, treatment of established infections with antibiotics, and correction of trichiasis before patients become blind. Because people with trichiasis are at most immediate risk of developing trachomatous visual impairment, surgery is the intervention that should be undertaken most urgently in trachoma-endemic areas. The acronym 'SAFE', used to encapsulate the trachoma control strategy recommended by the WHO, places the four elements of control in order of their priority: **S**urgery for trichiasis, **A**ntibiotics to reduce the prevalence of infection, and **F**ace washing and **E**nvironmental improvement to reduce transmission.

SURGERY

Surgical treatment of trichiasis aims to stop abrasion of the cornea by in-turned lashes, and thereby minimise on-going deterioration in vision. Many techniques have been described. Tarsal plate rotation (in which a transverse incision is made through the tarsus a few millimetres from the lid margin, and sutured under moderate tension so as to evert the lashes) is the best approach, with an estimated 77% success at 21 months after surgery.[27,28] Comparable results seem to be obtained regardless of whether the incision is full thickness (bilamellar tarsal rotation) or spares the skin of the lid (posterior lamellar tarsal rotation). Tarsal plate rotation is a simple, rapid procedure which can be performed effectively by ophthalmic nurses and ophthalmic medical assistants. This is fortunate, since in Africa, for example, there is only one ophthalmologist for every million people.

Traditional treatment for trichiasis often consists of mechanical epilation of ingrowing lashes using home-made forceps. Some control programmes recommend this to patients with minor trichiasis. Surgery, however, may be the better strategy, particularly because of the difficulties involved in monitoring disease progression in patients living in remote communities.[29]

Achieving high uptake of surgical services often proves difficult. Many programmes report that less than 50% of those offered correction of trichiasis actually present for surgery, even when transport to the health facility is provided by the programme and operations are performed free of charge. Village-based surgery, which has been shown to produce good operative outcomes,[30] may improve uptake by saving time for the patient and reducing fear of the procedure.[31]

ANTIBIOTICS

The recommended treatment for active trachoma is 1% tetracycline eye ointment, applied to both eyes twice daily for 6 weeks. However, tetracycline is difficult and often messy to self-administer, and stings on application; most individuals given treatment do not feel ill. As a result, compliance with tetracycline eye ointment is thought to be poor.

The demonstration that a single dose of 20 mg/kg oral azithromycin (to a maximum of 1 g) is at least as effective as prolonged courses of topical tetracycline[32] was, therefore, an exciting development. Under operational conditions, in which tetracycline is given to patients or their parents for application at home, single dose azithromycin is more effective, especially for severe active trachoma (TI).[33] Additionally, azithromycin is extremely well tolerated.

When antibiotics are given only to those with clinical signs of active trachoma, re-infection is likely to be rapid. Therefore, in areas in which the prevalence of TF in children is 10% or greater, the WHO recommends mass treatment (distribution of antibiotics to all residents).[34] Recent investigations show that the highest ocular *C. trachomatis* loads are found in children aged less than 5 years:[25] ensuring high antibiotic coverage in this age group may be critical to the success of trachoma control programmes.

At present, there are no good data demonstrating the relative effect of different frequencies of antibiotic distribution. Mathematical models suggest that in areas where trachoma is moderately endemic, annual treatment should be undertaken, but that in hyperendemic areas (prevalence of TF in children > 50%), treatment every 6 months may be required.[35] Trials to test this hypothesis are currently in progress. In the meantime, antibiotics should be distributed every 12 months. The WHO recommends that, once a decision has been taken to distribute antibiotics in an area, three annual treatments should be undertaken before re-assessment of disease prevalence to determine whether or not there is a need to continue.

Concerns have been raised that mass distribution of antibiotics, particularly azithromycin, will have an adverse impact on the antimicrobial resistance profiles of *C. trachomatis* and other human pathogens. There are at present no published data examining the effect of azithromycin on the antibiotic resistance profile of ocular *C. trachomatis* isolates. Surveillance seems warranted. A short-lived increase in the prevalence of macrolide resistance in nasopharyngeal isolates of *Streptococcus pneumoniae* was noted following the use of azithromycin against trachoma in Australia.[36] Larger studies in Nepal[37] and Tanzania,[38] however, suggest that multiple rounds of treatment may be required to affect antimicrobial resistance patterns in *S. pneumoniae* if background macrolide resistance is rare.

Some countries are fortunate to receive donations of azithromycin for trachoma control from the International Trachoma Initiative (ITI). Where azithromycin is not yet available or affordable, tetracycline remains the first-line treatment.

FACE WASHING

Because dirty faces are associated with active trachoma, West and colleagues undertook a community-randomised intervention trial to examine the impact of promoting face washing as an adjunct to mass treatment with tetracycline eye ointment. Three pairs of hyperendemic villages matched on maternal education and baseline prevalences of clean faces and active trachoma in young children were enrolled. Every resident of both intervention and control villages was offered topical tetracycline once daily for 30 days. In intervention villages, an intensive 1-month participatory campaign was conducted to encourage washing of children's faces. The prevalence of active trachoma in children was reduced following antibiotic treatment in both the intervention and control villages, but was returning towards pre-treatment levels by 12 months. In two of three intervention villages, the post-antibiotic increase in the prevalence of severe trachoma was slower than in their control pair. Whilst the face washing promotion campaign had no effect on the prevalence of TF, the proportion of children with sustained clean faces at follow-up was higher in the intervention group (35%) than the control group (26%), and clean faces were protective against both TF and TI.[39] In the majority of trachoma control programmes, however, resources to conduct health promotion campaigns of similar intensity at national level are unavailable. Cost-effective ways to convince water-insecure populations to use more of that water to keep faces clean are yet to be discovered.

ENVIRONMENTAL IMPROVEMENT

There is general agreement that improvements in a community's standard of living are associated with a decrease in trachoma transmission. Socio-economic development and increased living standards are believed to be responsible for the disappearance of trachoma from Europe and North America in the 20th century.

Unfortunately, merely waiting for socio-economic development to take place in trachoma-endemic areas will not prevent trachoma blindness. Proposed interventions include fly control through increased provision and use of latrines, improving access to water for face washing, and health education. Control of flies by regular ultra-low volume spraying of insecticide has proven effective in reducing the incidence of new cases of active trachoma in The Gambia.[26,40] However, insecticide spraying is unlikely to be sustainable in the long term. Because *M. sorbens* preferentially deposits its eggs on human faeces left exposed on the soil, provision of latrines could potentially be both effective and sustainable, but has not yet been shown to have a significant impact on disease.[40] No randomised controlled trials examining the effect of either health education or water provision have yet been published. Further work is required.

Key points for clinical practice

- Trachoma is the second most important cause of blindness. Trachoma blindness results from opacification of the cornea, which is due to corneal trauma produced by trichiasis. Trachomatous trichiasis develops only after many years of repeated conjunctival infection with ocular serovars of *Chlamydia trachomatis*.

- Trachoma blindness is eminently preventable, but is not curable.

- To be successful in reducing the incidence of trachoma blindness, prevention and control activities must be undertaken at the community level. Therefore, recognition of clinical signs of trachoma in patients attending paediatric clinics should be followed by discussions with ophthalmological colleagues and, in due course, formal assessment of the community prevalence of trachoma.

- Assessment of an individual for trachoma requires only magnifying loupes, sunlight, and the ability to evert an eyelid.

- The World Health Organization's simplified grading scheme for trachoma is very useful for assessment of the community prevalence of trachoma. It was not designed for diagnosis in individual patients, in whom the full clinical picture should be considered, together with the family history and socio-economic circumstances.

- Individuals with trachomatous trichiasis need urgent eyelid surgery. Wherever possible, surgery should be offered by well-trained ophthalmic personnel, in the patient's own community, at little or no cost to the patient.

- Appropriate antibiotics should be offered to patients with clinical signs of active trachoma, and all residents of any

(continued on next page)

(continued from previous page)

community in which the prevalence of follicular trachoma (TF) in children aged 1–9 years is 10% or more. There are two appropriate antibiotic regimens: one oral dose of azithromycin 20 mg/kg (or an equivalent height-based dose) to a maximum of 1 g, or tetracycline eye ointment applied to both eyes twice daily for 6 weeks. Communities that qualify for mass treatment should be given three annual rounds of treatment before re-assessment as to the need to continue.

- Health education to encourage face-washing, improved access to water, and improved access to and use of latrines, while not well supported by available trial data, are interventions that are likely to have great effect in the long term.

- Residents of trachoma-endemic communities must be involved in the assessment of disease burden and planning of control activities.

- The World Health Organization and its partners plan to eliminate trachoma as a public health problem by the year 2020.

ACKNOWLEDGEMENTS

We thank the International Trachoma Initiative, the Wellcome Trust – Burroughs Wellcome Fund, the Medical Research Council and the Edna McConnell Clark Foundation for supporting our research on trachoma.

References

1. Halberstaedter L, von Prowazek S. Über zelleinschlüsse parasitärer nature beim trachom. *Arb Gesundh Amte* 1907; **26**: 44–47.
2. T'ang FF, Chang HL, Huang YT, Wang KC. Studies on the etiology of trachoma with special reference to isolation of the virus in chick embryo. *Chin Med J (Engl)* 1957; **75**: 429–447.
3. Stephens RS, Kalman S, Lammel C *et al*. Genome sequence of an obligate intracellular pathogen of humans: *Chlamydia trachomatis*. *Science* 1998; **282**: 754–759.
4. Caldwell HD, Wood H, Crane D *et al*. Polymorphisms in *Chlamydia trachomatis* tryptophan synthase genes differentiate between genital and ocular isolates. *J Clin Invest* 2003; **111**: 1757–1769.
5. Grayston JT, Wang SP, Yeh LJ, Kuo CC. Importance of reinfection in the pathogenesis of trachoma. *Rev Infect Dis* 1985; **7**: 717–725.
6. Whittum-Hudson JA, Taylor HR, Farazdaghi M, Prendergast RA. Immunohistochemical study of the local inflammatory response to chlamydial ocular infection. *Invest Ophthalmol Vis Sci* 1986; **27**: 64–69.
7. al-Rajhi AA, Hidayat A, Nasr A, al-Faran M. The histopathology and the mechanism of entropion in patients with trachoma. *Ophthalmology* 1993; **100**: 1293–1296.
8. Bailey R, Duong T, Carpenter R, Whittle H, Mabey D. The duration of human ocular *Chlamydia trachomatis* infection is age dependent. *Epidemiol Infect* 1999; **123**: 479–486.
9. Williams DM, Grubbs BG, Pack E, Kelly K, Rank RG. Humoral and cellular immunity in secondary infection due to murine *Chlamydia trachomatis*. *Infect Immun* 1997; **65**: 2876–2882.
10. Bailey RL, Kajbaf M, Whittle HC, Ward ME, Mabey DC. The influence of local

anticlamydial antibody on the acquisition and persistence of human ocular chlamydial infection: IgG antibodies are not protective. *Epidemiol Infect* 1993; **111**: 315–324.

11. Bailey RL, Holland MJ, Whittle HC, Mabey DC. Subjects recovering from human ocular chlamydial infection have enhanced lymphoproliferative responses to chlamydial antigens compared with those of persistently diseased controls. *Infect Immun* 1995; **63**: 389–392.

12. Holland MJ, Bailey RL, Hayes LJ, Whittle HC, Mabey DC. Conjunctival scarring in trachoma is associated with depressed cell-mediated immune responses to chlamydial antigens. *J Infect Dis* 1993; **168**: 1528–1531.

13. Mabey DC, Bailey RL, Dunn D *et al*. Expression of MHC class II antigens by conjunctival epithelial cells in trachoma: implications concerning the pathogenesis of blinding disease. *J Clin Pathol* 1991; **44**: 285–289.

14. Morrison RP, Lyng K, Caldwell HD. Chlamydial disease pathogenesis. Ocular hypersensitivity elicited by a genus-specific 57-kDa protein. *J Exp Med* 1989; **169**: 663–675.

15. Peeling RW, Bailey RL, Conway DJ *et al*. Antibody response to the 60-kDa chlamydial heat-shock protein is associated with scarring trachoma. *J Infect Dis* 1998; **177**: 256–259.

16. Belland RJ, Scidmore MA, Crane DD *et al*. *Chlamydia trachomatis* cytotoxicity associated with complete and partial cytotoxin genes. *Proc Natl Acad Sci USA* 2001; **98**: 13984–13989.

17. Zhong G, Fan T, Liu L. Chlamydia inhibits interferon gamma-inducible major histocompatibility complex class II expression by degradation of upstream stimulatory factor 1. *J Exp Med* 1999; **189**: 1931–1938.

18. Mabey DC, Bailey RL, Ward ME, Whittle HC. A longitudinal study of trachoma in a Gambian village: implications concerning the pathogenesis of chlamydial infection. *Epidemiol Infect* 1992; **108**: 343–351.

19. Bobo LD, Novak N, Munoz B, Hsieh YH, Quinn TC, West S. Severe disease in children with trachoma is associated with persistent *Chlamydia trachomatis* infection. *J Infect Dis* 1997; **176**: 1524–1530.

20. West SK, Munoz B, Mkocha H, Hsieh YH, Lynch MC. Progression of active trachoma to scarring in a cohort of Tanzanian children. *Ophthalmic Epidemiol* 2001; **8**: 137–144.

21. Conway DJ, Holland MJ, Campbell AE *et al*. HLA class I and II polymorphisms and trachomatous scarring in a *Chlamydia trachomatis*-endemic population. *J Infect Dis* 1996; **174**: 643–646.

22. Conway DJ, Holland MJ, Bailey RL *et al*. Scarring trachoma is associated with polymorphism in the tumor necrosis factor alpha (TNF-alpha) gene promoter and with elevated TNF-alpha levels in tear fluid. *Infect Immun* 1997; **65**: 1003–1006.

23. Thylefors B, Dawson CR, Jones BR, West SK, Taylor HR. A simple system for the assessment of trachoma and its complications. *Bull World Health Organ* 1987; **65**: 477–483.

24. Thylefors B, Negrel AD, Pararajasegaram R, Dadzie KY. Global data on blindness. *Bull World Health Organ* 1995; **73**: 115–121.

25. Solomon AW, Holland MJ, Burton MJ *et al*. Strategies for control of trachoma: observational study with quantitative PCR. *Lancet* 2003; **362**: 198–204.

26. Emerson PM, Lindsay SW, Walraven GE *et al*. Effect of fly control on trachoma and diarrhoea [see comments]. *Lancet* 1999; **353**: 1401–1403.

27. Reacher MH, Munoz B, Alghassany A, Daar AS, Elbualy M, Taylor HR. A controlled trial of surgery for trachomatous trichiasis of the upper lid. *Arch Ophthalmol* 1992; **110**: 667–674.

28. Reacher MH, Huber MJ, Canagaratnam R, Alghassany A. A trial of surgery for trichiasis of the upper lid from trachoma. *Br J Ophthalmol* 1990; **74**: 109–113.

29. Bowman RJ, Faal H, Myatt M *et al*. Longitudinal study of trachomatous trichiasis in The Gambia. *Br J Ophthalmol* 2002; **86**: 339–343.

30. Bog H, Yorston D, Foster A. Results of community-based eyelid surgery for trichiasis due to trachoma. *Br J Ophthalmol* 1993; **77**: 81–83.

31. Bowman RJ, Soma OS, Alexander N *et al*. Should trichiasis surgery be offered in the village? A community randomised trial of village vs. health centre-based surgery. *Trop Med Int Health* 2000; **5**: 528–533.

32. Bailey RL, Arullendran P, Whittle HC, Mabey DC. Randomised controlled trial of single-dose azithromycin in treatment of trachoma. *Lancet* 1993; **342**: 453–456.

33. Bowman RJ, Sillah A, Van Dehn C *et al.* Operational comparison of single-dose azithromycin and topical tetracycline for trachoma. *Invest Ophthalmol Vis Sci* 2000; **41**: 4074–4079.

34. Schachter J, West SK, Mabey D *et al.* Azithromycin in control of trachoma. *Lancet* 1999; **354**: 630–635.

35. Lietman T, Porco T, Dawson C, Blower S. Global elimination of trachoma: how frequently should we administer mass chemotherapy? *Nat Med* 1999; **5**: 572–576.

36. Leach AJ, Shelby-James TM, Mayo M *et al.* A prospective study of the impact of community-based azithromycin treatment of trachoma on carriage and resistance of *Streptococcus pneumoniae*. *Clin Infect Dis* 1997; **24**: 356–362.

37. Fry AM, Jha HC, Lietman TM *et al.* Adverse and beneficial secondary effects of mass treatment with azithromycin to eliminate blindness due to trachoma in Nepal. *Clin Infect Dis* 2002; **35**: 395–402.

38. Batt SL, Charalambous BM, Solomon AW *et al.* Impact of azithromycin administration for trachoma control on the carriage of antibiotic-resistant *Streptococcus pneumoniae*. *Antimicrob Agents Chemother* 2003; **47**: 2765–2769.

39. West S, Munoz B, Lynch M *et al.* Impact of face-washing on trachoma in Kongwa, Tanzania. *Lancet* 1995; **345**: 155–158.

40. Emerson PM, Lindsay SW, Alexander N *et al.* Role of flies and provision of latrines in trachoma control: cluster-randomised controlled trial. *Lancet* 2004; **363**: 1093–1098.

Timothy J. David

Paediatric literature review – 2003

ALLERGY AND IMMUNOLOGY

ALLERGY

Clark AT *et al.* Food allergy in childhood. Arch Dis Child 2003; 88: 79–81. *Claims the danger has been underestimated.*

Clark AT *et al.* Interpretation of tests for nut allergy in one thousand patients, in relation to allergy or tolerance. Clin Exp Allergy 2003; 33: 1041–1045. *One cannot predict clinical reactivity from results in a wide 'grey area' of positive skin tests 3–7 mm; 22% of negative serum IgE tests are falsely re-assuring and 40% of positive serum IgE tests are misleading.*

Fiocchi A *et al.* Clinical tolerance to lactose in children with cow's milk allergy. Pediatrics 2003; 112: 359–362. *Children hypersensitivity to cow's milk are clinically tolerant to lactose.*

Fleischer DM *et al.* The natural progression of peanut allergy: resolution and the possibility of recurrence. J Allergy Clin Immunol 2003; 112: 183–189. *A subset of a highly selected sample of patients grew out of their allergy.*

Kagan RS *et al.* Prevalence of peanut allergy in primary-school children in Montreal, Canada. J Allergy Clin Immunol 2003; 112: 1223–1228. *Prevalence exceeds 1.0%. See also pp. 1203–1207.*

Latcham F *et al.* A consistent pattern of minor immunodeficiency and subtle enteropathy in children with multiple food allergy. J Pediatr 2003; 143: 39–47. *Describes a non IgE-mediated form of food allergy. See also pp. 7–9.*

Timothy J. David MD PhD FRCP FRCPCH DCH
Professor, Booth Hall Children's Hospital, Charlestown Road, Blackley, Manchester M9 7AA, UK
Tel: +44 161 220 5536; Fax: +44 161 904 9320; E-mail: t.david@netcomuk.co.uk

Leung DYM *et al.* Effect of anti-IgE therapy in patients with peanut allergy. N Engl J Med 2003; 348: 986–993. *Substantially increases the threshold of sensitivity.*

Maleki SJ *et al.* The major peanut allergen, ara h 2, functions as a trypsin inhibitor, and roasting enhances this function. J Allergy Clin Immunol 2003; 112: 190–195. *Roasting enhances allergenic properties.*

Pumphrey RS. Fatal posture in anaphylactic shock. J Allergy Clin Immunol 2003; 112: 451–452. *Treatment of anaphylaxis should include lying flat and elevation of legs to assist venous return.*

Radcliffe MJ *et al.* Enzyme potentiated desensitisation in treatment of seasonal allergic rhinitis: double blind randomised controlled study. BMJ 2003; 327: 251–254. *No benefit.*

Simonte SJ *et al.* Relevance of casual contact with peanut butter in children with peanut allergy. J Allergy Clin Immunol 2003; 112: 180–182. *Skin contact and inhalation did not cause systemic or respiratory reactions.*

COMMUNITY

Gillberg C *et al.* Learning disability. Lancet 2003; 362: 811–821. *Review.*

Nikolopoulou M *et al.* Preventing sleeping problems in infants who are at risk of developing them. Arch Dis Child 2003; 88: 108–111. *Behavioural programme might help.*

Weitoft GR *et al.* Mortality, severe morbidity, and injury in children living with single parents in Sweden: a population-based study. Lancet 2003; 361: 289–295. *Children of single parents have increased risks of mortality, severe morbidity and injury.*

Whitehead M *et al.* What puts children of lone parents at a health disadvantage? Lancet 2003; 361: 271. *Editorial.*

ACCIDENTS

Agran PF *et al.* Rates of pediatric injuries by 3-month intervals for children 0 to 3 years of age. Pediatrics 2003; 111: e683–e692. *Children aged 15 to 17 months had the highest overall injury rate before age 15 years.*

Brehaut JC *et al.* Childhood behaviour disorders and injuries among children and youth: a population-based study. Pediatrics 2003; 111: 262–269. *Small increase in risk of injury.*

Bull MJ *et al.* Poison treatment in the home. Pediatrics 2003; 112: 1182–1185. *Review.*

Bull MJ *et al.* Prevention of drowning in infants, children, and adolescents. Pediatrics 2003; 112: 437–445. *Policy statement.*

Garros D *et al.* Strangulation with intravenous tubing: a previously undescribed adverse advent in children. Pediatrics 2003; 111: e732–e734. *2 cases.*

Kendrick D *et al*. Inequalities in cycle helmet use: cross sectional survey in schools in deprived areas of Nottingham. Arch Dis Child 2003; 88: 876–880. *Half the children owned a helmet but only 29% of these always wore their helmet.*

Lee AJ *et al*. Cycle helmets. Arch Dis Child 2003; 88: 465–466. *Review.*

Maconochie I. Accident prevention. Arch Dis Child 2003; 88: 275–277. *Review.*

Parkinson GW *et al*. Bicycle helmet assessment during well visits reveals severe shortcomings in condition and fit. Pediatrics 2003; 112: 320–323. *96% of children wore helmets in inadequate condition and/or with inadequate fit.*

Pickett W *et al*. Injuries experienced by infant children: a population-based epidemiological analysis. Pediatrics 2003; 111: e365–e370. *Leading causes of injury were falls, ingestion injuries and burns.*

Ratnapalan S *et al*. Measuring a toddler's mouthful: toxicological considerations. J Pediatr 2003; 142: 729–730. *Mean volume was 9.3 ml.*

Skellett S *et al*. Immobilisation of the cervical spine in children. BMJ 2002; 324: 591-593. *Failure to immobilise is commonplace.*

Titus M *et al*. Accidental scald burns in sinks. Pediatrics 2003; 111: e191–e194. *Report of 3 cases.*

Tonkin S *et al*. Simple car seat insert to prevent upper airway narrowing in preterm infants: a pilot study. Pediatrics 2003; 112: 907-913. *Flexion of the head on the body is a significant contributor to oxygen desaturation.*

CEREBRAL PALSY

Jarvis S *et al*. Cerebral palsy and intrauterine growth in single births: European collaborative study. Lancet 2003; 362: 1106–1111. *Risk rises when weight is well above normal as well as when it is well below normal. See also pp. 1089–1090.*

Nelson KB *et al*. Can we prevent cerebral palsy? N Engl J Med 2003; 349: 1765–1769. *Editorial.*

Rosenbaum P *et al*. Cerebral palsy: what parents and doctors want to know. BMJ 2003; 326: 970–974. *Review.*

Worley G *et al*. Secondary sexual characteristics in children with cerebral palsy and moderate to severe motor impairment: a cross-sectional survey. Pediatrics 2002; 110: 897–902. *Puberty begins earlier but ends later in white children with cerebral palsy.*

CHILD ABUSE

Bariciak ED *et al*. Dating of bruises in children: an assessment of physician accuracy. Pediatrics 2003; 112: 804–807. *Large individual variability and poor inter-rater reliability.*

Black J *et al*. Child abuse by intentional iron poisoning presenting as shock and persistent acidosis. Pediatrics 2003; 111: 197–199. *Case report.*

Bonnier C *et al*. Neuroimaging of intraparenchymal lesions predicts outcome in shaken baby syndrome. Pediatrics 2003; 112: 808–814. *14 (61%) children had severe disabilities, 8 (35%) had moderate disabilities, and 1 (4%) was normal.*

Coulthard MG *et al*. Distinguishing between salt poisoning and hypernatraemic dehydration in children. BMJ 2003; 326: 157–160. *Review*.

DeRusso PA *et al*. Fractures in biliary atresia misinterpreted as child abuse. Pediatrics 2003; 112: 185–188. *Report of 3 cases*.

de San Lazaro C *et al*. Shaking infant trauma induced by misuse of a baby chair. Arch Dis Child 2003; 88: 632–634. *Suggests violent rocking in chair could injure baby*.

de Silva P *et al*. Physiological periostitis; a potential pitfall. Arch Dis Child 2003; 88: 1124–1125. *2 cases mistaken for abuse*.

Golden MH *et al*. How to distinguish between neglect and deprivational abuse. Arch Dis Child 2003; 88: 105–107. *Review*.

Hall D. Child protection – lessons from Victoria Climbie. BMJ 2003; 326: 293–294. *Editorial*.

Heppenstall-Heger A *et al*. Healing patterns in anogenital injuries: a longitudinal study of injuries associated with sexual abuse, accidental injuries, or genital surgery in the preadolescent child. Pediatrics 2003; 112: 182–837. *Anogenital trauma heals quickly, often without residua*.

Hettler J *et al*. Can the initial history predict whether a child with a head injury has been abused? Pediatrics 2003; 111: 602–607. *Having no history of trauma had a high specificity for abuse*.

Kemp AM *et al*. Apnoea and brain swelling in non-accidental head injury. Arch Dis Child 2003; 111: 602–607. *22/65 had apnoea on presentation*.

Kimberlin DW *et al*. Effect of ganciclovir therapy on hearing in symptomatic congenital cytomegalovirus disease involving the central nervous system: a randomized, controlled trial. J Pediatr 2003; 143: 16–25. *Prevents hearing deterioration at 6 months*.

Mandelstam SA *et al*. Complementary use of radiological skeletal survey and bone scintigraphy in detection of bony injuries in suspected child abuse. Arch Dis Child 2003; 88: 387–390. *Should both be performed in cases of suspected child abuse*.

Rubin DM *et al*. Occult head injury in high-risk abused children. Pediatrics 2003; 111: 1382–1386. *Risk factors include rib fractures, multiple fractures, facial injury, and younger age (< 6 months). One should proceed directly to CT or MRI in high-risk populations*.

Salter D *et al*. Development of sexually abusive behaviour in sexually victimised males: a longitudinal study. Lancet 2003; 361: 471–476. *Of 224 victims, 26 committed sexual offences. See also pp. 446–447*.

Schreier H. Munchausen by proxy defined. Pediatrics 2002; 110: 985–988. *Review*.

Southall DP *et al*. Classification of child abuse by motive and degree rather than type of injury. Arch Dis Child 2003; 88: 101–104. *Review*.

Stanton AN. Sudden unexpected death in infancy associated with maltreatment: evidence from long term follow up of siblings. Arch Dis Child 2003; 88: 699–701. *Out of 69, in only 2 did the circumstances suggest maltreatment*.

IMMUNISATION

Baker CJ *et al.* Group B streptococcal conjugate vaccines. Arch Dis Child 2003; 88: 375–378. *Review.*

Bohlke K *et al.* Risk of anaphylaxis after vaccination of children and adolescents. Pediatrics 2003; 112: 815–820. *A rare event.*

Bothamley GH *et al.* Tuberculin testing before BCG vaccination. BMJ 2003; 327: 243–244. *Editorial.*

Brisson M *et al.* Varicella vaccination in England and Wales: cost-utility analysis. Arch Dis Child 2003; 88: 862–869. *Routine infant varicella vaccination is unlikely to be cost-effective.*

Furth SL *et al.* Varicella vaccination in children with nephrotic syndrome: a report of the southwest pediatric nephrology study group. J Pediatr 2003; 142: 145–148. *Well tolerated and immunogenic, including in those on low-dose prednisone.*

Grant CC *et al.* Delayed immunisation and risk of pertussis in infants: unmatched case-control study. BMJ 2003; 326: 852–853. *Delayed immunisation is a specific risk factor for admission to hospital with pertussis.*

Heath PT *et al.* *Haemophilus influenzae* type b vaccine-booster campaign. BMJ 2003; 326: 1158–1159. *Editorial.*

Heath PT *et al.* Hib vaccination in infants born prematurely. Arch Dis Child 2003; 88: 206–210. *Affords a high level of protection.*

Makela A *et al.* Neurologic disorders after measles-mumps-rubella vaccination. Pediatrics 2002; 110: 957–963. *No association.*

Miller E *et al.* Bacterial infections, immune overload, and MMR vaccine. Arch Dis Child 2003; 88: 222–223. *No support for the concept of 'immunological overload'.*

Nelson KB *et al.* Thimerosal and autism? Pediatrics 2003; 111: 674–679. *Review.*

Offit PA *et al.* Addressing parents' concerns: do vaccines cause allergic or autoimmune disease? Pediatrics 2003; 111: 653–659. *Review.*

Pai VA *et al.* Influenza vaccine. Arch Dis Child 2003; 88: 665–665. *Questions the need in asthma and diabetes.*

Ramsay ME *et al.* Herd immunity from meningococcal serogroup C conjugate vaccination in England: database analysis. BMJ 2003; 326: 365–366. *Attack rate in unvaccinated population reduced.*

Saari TN *et al.* Immunisation of preterm and low birth weight infants. Pediatrics 2003; 112: 193–198. *Review.*

Steinhoff M *et al.* Conjugate Hib vaccines. Lancet 2003; 361: 360–361. *Editorial.*

INFANT FEEDING

Bhandari N *et al.* Effect of community-based promotion of exclusive breastfeeding on diarrhoeal illness and growth: a cluster randomised controlled trial. Lancet 2003; 361: 1418–1423. *Reduces the risk of diarrhoea, and does not lead to growth faltering.*

Carbajal R *et al.* Analgesic effect of breast feeding in term neonates: randomised controlled trial. BMJ 2003; 326: 13–15. *Effectively reduces response to pain.*

Foote KD *et al.* Weaning of infants. Arch Dis Child 2003; 88: 488–492. *Review.*

MacDonald PD *et al.* Neonatal weight loss in breast and formula fed infants. Arch Dis Child 2003; 88: F472–F476. *Early neonatal weight loss is defined, allowing identification of infants who merit closer assessment and support.*

Michie C *et al.* The challenge of mastitis. Arch Dis Child 2003; 88: 818–821. *Review.*

Read JS *et al.* Human milk, breastfeeding, and transmission of human immunodeficiency virus type 1 in the United States. Pediatrics 2003; 112: 1196–1205. *Review.*

SCREENING

Clarke MP *et al.* Randomised controlled trial of treatment of unilateral visual impairment detected at preschool vision screening. BMJ 2003; 327: 1251–1254. *Treatment is worthwhile in those with the poorest acuity.*

Dutton GN *et al.* Should we be screening for and treating amblyopia? BMJ 2003; 327: 1242–1243. *Editorial.*

Pass K. Not as pink as you think! Pediatrics 2003; 111: 670–671. *Editorial about screening for heart defects in newborns using pulse oximetry.*

Pirozzo S *et al.* Whispered voice test for screening for hearing impairment in adults and children: systematic review. BMJ 2003; 327: 967–970. *Simple and accurate test.*

SUDDEN INFANT DEATH SYNDROME (SIDS)

Blackman LR *et al.* Apnea, sudden infant death syndrome, and home monitoring. Pediatrics 2003; 111: 914–917. *American Academy of Pediatrics' policy statement.*

Jones KL *et al.* Vascular endothelial growth factor in the cerebrospinal fluid of infants who died of sudden infant death syndrome: evidence for antecedent hypoxia. Pediatrics 2003; 111: 358–363. *Hypoxia precedes sudden death.*

Platt MJ *et al.* The epidemiology of sudden infant death syndrome. Arch Dis Child 2003; 88: 27–29. *The crude relative risk of SIDS in twins is twice that in singletons.*

Wailoo M *et al.* Signs and symptoms of illness in early infancy: associations with sudden infant death. Arch Dis Child 2003; 88: 1001–1004. *No special pattern of symptoms was seen.*

DERMATOLOGY

Alston SJ *et al.* Persistent and recurrent tinea corporis in children treated with combination antifungal/corticosteroid agents. Pediatrics 2003; 111: 201–203. *Best to use single agent antifungal therapy.*

Balkrishnan R *et al.* Disease severity and associated family impact in childhood atopic dermatitis. Arch Dis Child 2003; 88: 423–427. *Perceived severity is the driver of the family impact of this condition.*

Fuller LC *et al.* Diagnosis and management of scalp ringworm. BMJ 2003; 326: 539–541. *Review.*

Leung DYM *et al.* Atopic dermatitis. Lancet 2003; 361: 151–160. *Review.*

Ramsay HM *et al.* Herbal creams used for atopic eczema in Birmingham, UK, illegally contain potent corticosteroids. Arch Dis Child 2003; 88: 1056–1057. *The majority of herbal creams analysed contained potent or very potent topical steroids.*

Warner M. Recent developments in lasers and the treatment of birthmarks. Arch Dis Child 2003; 88: 372–374. *Review.*

Williams HC. Evening primrose oil for atopic dermatitis. BMJ 2003; 327: 1358–1359. *Editorial. See also pp. 1385–1387.*

ENDOCRINOLOGY

Frias JL *et al.* Health supervision for children with Turner syndrome. Pediatrics 2003; 111: 692–702. *Review.*

Oerbeck B *et al.* Congenital hypothyroidism: influence of disease severity and L-thyroxine treatment on intellectual, motor, and school-associated outcomes in young adults. Pediatrics 2003; 112: 923–930. *Outcome was associated with severity, indicating a prenatal effect.*

DIABETES

Betts PR *et al.* Doctor, who will be looking after my child's diabetes? Arch Dis Child 2003; 88: 6–7. *Review of multidisciplinary team.*

Channon S *et al.* A pilot study of motivational interviewing in adolescents with diabetes. Arch Dis Child 2003; 88: 680–683. *May be useful.*

Jefferson IG *et al.* Diabetes services in the UK: third national survey confirms continuing deficiencies. Arch Dis Child 2003; 88: 53–56. *Shortage of specialist nurses and doctors.*

Ludvigsson J *et al.* Continuous subcutaneous glucose monitoring improved metabolic control in pediatric patients with Type 1 diabetes: a controlled crossover study. Pediatrics 2003; 111: 933–938. *A useful tool for education and control.*

Nordfeldt S *et al.* Prevention of severe hypoglycaemia in type 1 diabetes: a randomised controlled population study. Arch Dis Child 2003; 88: 240–245. *High quality video programmes and brochures may contribute to the prevention.*

Torrance T *et al.* Insulin pumps. Arch Dis Child 2003; 88: 949–953. *Review.*

Wills CJ *et al.* Retrospective review of care and outcomes in young adults with type 1 diabetes. BMJ 2003; 327: 260–261. *Glycaemic control is generally poor, attendance at the clinic and screening for complications are suboptimal, and microvascular complications are common.*

GROWTH

Argall JAW *et al*. A comparison of two commonly used methods of weight estimation. Arch Dis Child 2003; 88: 789–790. *The average weight of children is increasing.*

Diaz-Gomez NM *et al*. The effect of zinc supplementation on linear growth, body composition, and growth factors in preterm infants. Pediatrics 2003; 111: 1002–1009. *Positive effect.*

Lee PA *et al*. International small for gestational age advisory board consensus development conference statement: management of short children born small for gestational age, April 21 – October 1, 2001. Pediatrics 2003; 111: 1253–1261. *Review and recommendations.*

Lee PA *et al*. Persistent short stature, other potential outcomes, and the effect of growth hormone treatment in children who are born small for gestational age. Pediatrics 2003; 112: 1253–1261. *Review.*

OBESITY

Kaur H *et al*. Duration of television watching is associated with increased body mass index. J Pediatr 2003; 143: 506–511. *Television viewing leads to overweight.*

Li L *et al*. Breast feeding and obesity in childhood: cross sectional study. BMJ 2003; 327: 904–905. *No protection.*

Prentice AM *et al*. Intrauterine factors, adiposity, and hyperinsulinaemia. BMJ 2003; 327: 880–881. *Editorial.*

Wing YK *et al*. A controlled study of sleep related disorders breathing in obese children. Arch Dis Child 2003; 88: 1043–1047. *26–32% had sleep disordered breathing.*

ENT

Block SL. Acute otitis media: bunnies, disposables, and bacterial original sin! Pediatrics 2003; 111: 217–218. *Only nickel-cadmium or lithium battery-powered otoscopes should be used.*

Craig FW *et al*. Retropharyngeal abscess in children: clinical presentation, utility of imaging, and current management. Pediatrics 2003; 111: 1394–1398. *Review of 64 cases.*

Gray RF *et al*. Cochlear implantation for progressive hearing loss. Arch Dis Child 2003; 88: 708–711. *Report of 6 cases.*

Paradise JL *et al*. Otitis media and tympanostomy tube insertion during the first three years of life: developmental outcomes at the age of four years. Pediatrics 2003; 112: 265–277. *Developmental outcome not affected.*

Reefhuis J *et al*. Risk of bacterial meningitis in children with cochlear implants. N Engl J Med 2003; 349: 435–445. *Postimplantation bacterial meningitis was strongly associated with the use of an implant with a positioner.*

Ruohola A *et al*. Antibiotic treatment of acute otorrhea through tympanostomy tube: randomized double-blind placebo-controlled study with daily follow-up. Pediatrics 2003; 111: 1061–1067. *Significantly accelerates resolution.*

Veenhoven R *et al*. Effect of conjugate pneumococcal vaccine followed by polysaccharide pneumococcal vaccine on recurrent acute otitis media: a randomised study. Lancet 2003; 361: 2189–2195. *No benefit.*

GASTROENTEROLOGY

Chial HJ *et al*. Rumination syndrome in children and adolescents: diagnosis, treatment and prognosis. Pediatrics 2003; 111: 158–162. *Effortless regurgitation into the mouth of recently ingested food followed by rechewing and reswallowing or expulsion.*

Moore DJ *et al*. Double-blind placebo-controlled trial of omeprazole in irritable infants with gastroesophageal reflux. J Pediatr 2003; 143: 219–223. *Omeprazole significantly reduced oesophageal acid exposure but not irritability. See also pp. 147–148.*

Salvatore S *et al*. Gastroesophageal reflux and cow milk allergy: is there a link? Pediatrics 2003; 110: 972–984. *Review.*

Sawczenko A *et al*. Presenting features of inflammatory bowel disease in Great Britain and Ireland 2003; 88: 995–1000. *Median delay from onset of symptoms to diagnosis was 5 months.*

Wenzl TG *et al*. Effects of thickened feeding on gastroesophageal reflux in infants: a placebo-controlled crossover study using intraluminal impedance. Pediatrics 2003; 111: e355–e359. *Carob bean gum is an efficient therapy.*

GENETICS AND MALFORMATIONS

GENETICS

Bailey DB *et al*. Discovering fragile X syndrome: family experiences and perceptions. Pediatrics 2003; 111: 407–416. *Review.*

Donnai D *et al*. How clinicians add to knowledge of development. Lancet 2003; 362: 477–484. *Review.*

Reynolds RM *et al*. Von Recklinghausen's neurofibromatosis: neurofibromatosis type 1. Lancet 2003; 361: 1552–1554. *Case report and review.*

MALFORMATIONS

Hall JG. Twinning. Lancet 2003; 362: 735–743. *Review.*

Rasmussen SA *et al*. Population-based analyses of mortality in trisomy 13 and trisomy 18. Lancet 2003; 111: 777–784. *5–10% survive beyond the first year of life.*

Roizen NJ *et al*. Down's syndrome. Lancet 2003; 361: 1081–1289. *Review.*

HAEMATOLOGY

Bolton-Maggs PHB *et al*. Haemophilias A and B. Lancet 2003; 361: 1801–1809. *Review.*

Claster S *et al*. Managing sickle cell disease. BMJ 2003; 327: 1151–1155. *Review.*

Hey E *et al*. Vitamin K – what, why, and when. Arch Dis Child 2003; 88: F80–F83. *Review.*

Kuhne T *et al*. A prospective comparative study of 2540 infants and children with newly diagnosed idiopathic thrombocytopenic purpura (ITP) from the intercontinental childhood ITP study group. J Pediatr 2003; 143: 605–608. *Study of 2540 patients.*

Lykavieris P *et al*. Bleeding tendency in children with Alagille syndrome. Pediatrics 2003; 111: 167–170. *The mechanism of the bleding is unclear.*

Pereira SP *et al*. Intestinal absorption of mixed micellar phylloquinone (vitamin K) is unreliable in infants with conjugated hyperbilirubinaemia: implications for oral prophylaxis of vitamin K deficiency bleeding. Arch Dis Child 2003; 88: F113–F118. *Explanation for the failure of some oral vitamin K regimens.*

Rayment R *et al*. Neonatal alloimmune thrombocytopenia. BMJ 2003; 327: 331–332. *Report of 3 cases.*

Vorstman EBA *et al*. Brain haemorrhage in five infants with coagulopathy. Arch Dis Child 2003; 88: 1119–1121. *Report of 5 cases.*

INFECTIOUS DISEASE

Abrams EJ. Should treatment be started among all HIV-infected children and then stopped? Lancet 2003; 362: 1595–1596. *Editorial. See also pp. 1605–1611.*

Balasegaram S *et al*. A decade of change: tuberculosis in England and Wales 1988–98. Arch Dis Child 2003; 88: 772–777. *From 1988 to 1998 there was no major change in the overall rate of disease in children.*

Banatvala JE *et al*. Rubella. Lancet 2003; 363: 1127–1137. *Review.*

Bashir HE *et al*. Diagnosis and treatment of bacterial meningitis. Arch Dis Child 2003; 88: 615–620. *Review.*

Blutt SE *et al*. Rotavirus antigenaemia and viraemia: a common event. Lancet 2003; 362: 1445–1449. *Antigen was present in 22 of 33 serum samples.*

Bochud PY *et al*. Pathogenesis of sepsis: new concepts and implications for future treatment. BMJ 2003; 326: 262–266. *Review.*

Crowcroft NS *et al*. Severe and unrecognised: pertussis in UK infants. Arch Dis Child 2003; 88: 802–806. *Severe pertussis is under diagnosed and may co-exist with RSV infection.*

Davison KL *et al*. The epidemiology of acute meningitis in children in England and Wales. Arch Dis Child 2003; 88: 662–664. *Review.*

Duke T *et al.* Measles: not just another viral exanthem. Lancet 2003; 361: 763–773. *Review.*

Halket S *et al.* Long term follow up after meningitis in infancy: behaviour of teenagers. Arch Dis Child 2003; 88: 395–398. *Is worse than that of control children.*

Havens PL. Postexposure prophylaxis in children and adolescents for nonoccupational exposure to human immunodeficiency virus. Pediatrics 2003; 111: 1475–1489. *Review.*

Loveland J *et al.* Bowel obstruction in an infant with AIDS. Arch Dis Child 2003; 88: 825–826. *Case report.*

Modlin JF *et al.* Case 25-2003: a newborn boy with petechiae and thrombocytopenia. N Engl J Med 2003; 349: 691–700. *Case of congenital thrombocytopaenia.*

Pathan N *et al.* Pathophysiology of meningococcal meningitis and septicaemia. Arch Dis Child 2003; 88: 601–607. *Review.*

Saez-Llorens X *et al.* Bacterial meningitis in children. Lancet 2003; 361: 2139–2148. *Review.*

Stanley SL *et al.* Amoebiasis. Lancet 2003; 361: 1025–1034. *Review.*

Sticker T *et al.* Vulvovaginitis in prepubertal girls. Arch Dis Child 2003; 88: 324–326. *Pathogenic bacteria were isolated in 36% of cases.*

Stringer JSA *et al.* Nevirapine to prevent mother to child transmission of HIV-1 among women of unknown serostatus. Lancet 2003; 362: 1850–1853. *Review.*

Thomas A *et al.* National guideline for the management of suspected sexually transmitted infections in children and young people. Arch Dis Child 2002; 78: 324–331. *Review.*

Welch SB *et al.* Treatment of meningococcal infection. Arch Dis Child 2003; 88: 608–614. *Review.*

West NS *et al.* Fever in returned travellers: a prospective review of hospital admissions for a 2.5 year period. Arch Dis Child 2003; 88: 432–434. *Diarrhoeal illness and malaria were the most common diagnoses.*

MEDICINE IN THE TROPICS

Bhan MK *et al.* Management of the severely malnourished child: perspective from developing countries. BMJ 2003; 326: 146–151. *Review.*

Duke T *et al.* Chloramphenicol or ceftriaxone, or both, as treatment for meningitis in developing countries? Arch Dis Child 2003; 88: 536–539. *Highlights the urgent need to reduce the costs of third-generation cephalosporins.*

Grotto I *et al.* Vitamin A supplementation and childhood morbidity from diarrhea and respiratory infections: a meta-analysis. J Pediatr 2003; 142: 297–304. *Should be offered only to individuals or populations with vitamin A deficiency.*

Molyneux EM *et al.* The effect of HIV infection on paediatric bacterial meningitis in Blantyre, Malawi. Arch Dis Child 2003; 88: 1112–1118. *High mortality and prone to recurrent disease.*

Rahmathullah L *et al.* Impact of supplementing newborn infants with vitamin A on early infant mortality: community based randomised trial in southern India. BMJ 2003; 88: 254–257. *Review.*

Waterston J *et al.* Monitoring the marketing of infant formula feeds. BMJ 2003; 326: 113–114. *Editorial. See also pp. 137–130.*

METABOLIC

Krebs NF *et al.* Prevention of pediatric overweight and obesity. Pediatrics 2003; 112: 424–430. *Policy statement.*

Mehta A *et al.* Transient hyperinsulinism associated with macrosomia, hypertrophic obstructive cardiomyopathy, hepatomegaly, and nephromegaly. Arch Dis Child 2003; 88: 822–824. *Case report.*

Oginni LM *et al.* Radiological and biochemical resolution of nutritional rickets with calcium. Arch Dis Child 2003; 88: 812–817. *Calcium supplementation alone effected healing of rickets in most children.*

Reilly JJ *et al.* Health consequences of obesity. Arch Dis Child 2003; 88: 748–752. *Review.*

Selzer RR *et al.* Adverse effect of nitrous oxide in a child with 5, 10-methylene-tetrahydrofolate reductase deficiency. N Engl J Med 2003; 349: 45–50. *Case report.*

Singh J *et al.* The investigation of hypocalcaemia and rickets. Arch Dis Child 2003; 88: 403–407. *Review.*

Speiser PW *et al.* Congenital adrenal hyperplasia. N Engl J Med 2003; 349: 776–788. *Review.*

MISCELLANEOUS

Berde C *et al.* Pain, anxiety, distress, and suffering: interrelated, but not interchangeable. J Pediatr 2003; 142: 361–363. *Editorial.*

Black RE *et al.* Where and why are 10 million children dying every year. Lancet 2003; 361: 2226–2234. *Review.*

Blum NJ *et al.* Relationship between age at initiation of toilet training and duration of training: a prospective study. Pediatrics 2003; 111: 810–814. *Useful research data.*

Breau LM *et al.* Relation between pain and self-injurious behaviour in nonverbal children with severe cognitive impairments. J Pediatr 2003; 142: 498–503. *Children with severe cognitive impairments who self injure do not have reduced pain expression.*

Brook I *et al*. Unexplained fever in young children: how to manage severe bacterial infection. BMJ 2003; 327: 1094–1097. *Review*.

Bryce J *et al*. Reducing child mortality: can public health deliver? Lancet 2003; 362: 159–164. *Review*.

Chow LML *et al*. Peripherally inserted central catheter (PICC) fracture and embolization in the pediatric population. J Pediatr 2003; 142: 141–144. *Sufficiently common to warrant mentioning when obtaining informed consent.*

Dalton MA *et al*. Effect of viewing smoking in movies on adolescent smoking initiation: a cohort study. Lancet 2003; 362: 281–285. *Promotes smoking initiation. See also pp. 258–259.*

Durward A *et al*. Hypoalbuminaemia in critically ill children: incidence, prognosis, and influence on the anion gap. Arch Dis Child 2003; 88: 419–422. *Common but not an independent predictor of mortality.*

Eccleston C *et al*. Managing chronic pain in children and adolescents. BMJ 2003; 326: 1408–1409. *Editorial.*

Forjuoh SN *et al*. Parental knowledge of school backpack weight and contents. Arch Dis Child 2003; 88: 18–19. *The majority of parents whose children's backpacks weigh 10% or more of their body weights, do not know the backpack weights or contents. See also Pediatrics 2003; 111: 163–166.*

Frush DP *et al*. Computed tomography and radiation risks: what pediatric health care providers should know. Pediatrics 2003; 112: 951–957. *Review. See also pp. 971–973.*

Gillespie D *et al*. Knowledge into action for child survival. Lancet 2003; 362: 323–327. *Review.*

Hofhuis W *et al*. Adverse health effects of prenatal and postnatal tobacco smoke exposure on children. Arch Dis Child 2003; 88: 1086–1090. *Review.*

Jones G *et al*. How many child deaths can we prevent this year? Lancet 2003; 362: 65–71. *Review.*

Kaplan DW *et al*. Identifying and treating eating disorders. Pediatrics 2003; 111: 204–211. *Review.*

Klass PE *et al*. The developing brain and early learning. Arch Dis Child 2003; 88: 651–654. *Review.*

Li J *et al*. Mortality in parents after death of a child in Denmark: a nationwide follow-up study. Lancet 2003; 361: 363–367. *Increased mortality.*

Mrdjenovic G *et al*. Nutritional and energetic consequences of sweetened drink consumption in 6 to 13 year old children. J Pediatr 2003; 142: 604–610. *Excessive sweetened drink consumption is associated with higher daily energy intake and greater weight gain.*

Mrusek S *et al*. Henoch-Schonlein purpura. Lancet 2003; 363: 1116–1116. *Florid atypical case.*

Nigrovic PA *et al*. Raynaud's phenomenon in children: a retrospective review of 123 patients. Pediatrics 2003; 111: 715–721. *Principally affects girls and frequently free of association with connective tissue disease.*

Persing J *et al.* Prevention and management of positional skull deformities in infants. Pediatrics 2003; 112: 199–202. *Review.*

Ramnarayan P *et al.* Does the use of a specialised paediatric retrieval service result in the loss of vital stabilisation skills among referring hospital staff? Arch Dis Child 2003; 88: 851–854. *No.*

Sundel RP *et al.* Corticosteroids in the initial treatment of Kawasaki disease: report of a randomized trial. J Pediatr 2003; 142: 611–616. *Resulted in faster resolution of fever.*

Zulian F *et al.* Acute surgical abdomen as presenting manifestation of Kawasaki disease. J Pediatr 2003; 142: 731–735. *10 of 219 patients presented with acute abdomen.*

NEONATOLOGY

Alkalay AL *et al.* Hemodynamic changes in anemic premature infants: are we allowing the hematocrits to fall too low? Pediatrics 2003; 112: 838–845. *Apparently 'stable' anaemic infants may be in a clinically unrecognised high cardiac output state.*

Allwood ACL *et al.* Changes in resuscitation practice at birth. Arch Dis Child 2003; 88: F375–F379. *Rate of intubation and ventilation fell.*

Askie LM *et al.* Oxygen-saturation targets and outcomes in extremely preterm infants. N Engl J Med 2003; 349: 959–967. *No benefit of higher oxygen-saturation range.*

Bar-Oz B *et al.* Comparison of meconium and neonatal hair analysis for detection of gestational exposure to drugs of abuse. Arch Dis Child 2003; 88: F98–F100. *Meconium may be more sensitive, but neonatal hair is available for 3 months.*

Battin MR *et al.* Treatment of term infants with head cooling and mild systemic hypothermia (35.0°C and 34.5°C) after perinatal asphyxia. Pediatrics 2003; 111: 244–251. *A stable, well-tolerated method.*

Beardsall K *et al.* Pericardial effusion and cardiac tamponade as complications of neonatal long lines: are they really a problem? Arch Dis Child 2003; 88: F292–F295. *A serious but infrequent complication.*

Blackmon L *et al.* Controversies concerning vitamin K and the newborn. Pediatrics 2003; 112: 191–192. *American Academy of Pediatrics' policy statement.*

Chow LC *et al.* Can changes in clinical practice decrease the incidence of severe retinopathy of prematurity in very low birth weight infants? Pediatrics 2003; 111: 339–345. *Apparently yes.*

Cowan F *et al.* Origin and timing of brain lesions in term infants with neonatal encephalopathy. Lancet 2003; 361: 736–742. *Review.*

Dasgupta SJ *et al.* Hypotension in the very low birthweight infant: the old, the new, and the uncertain. Arch Dis Child 2003; 88: F450–F454. *Review.*

Debillon T *et al.* Limitations of ultrasonography for diagnosing white matter damage in preterm infants. Arch Dis Child 2003; 88: F275–F279. *Effective in detecting severe lesions.*

De Paoli AG *et al*. Nasal CPAP for neonates: what do we know in 2003? Arch Dis Child 2003; 88: F168–F172. *Review*.

Fowlie PW *et al*. Prophylactic indomethacin for preterm infants: a systematic review and meta-analysis. Arch Dis Child 2003; 88: F464–F466. *Short term benefits*.

Frey B *et al*. Oxygen administration in infants. Arch Dis Child 2003; 88: F84–F88. *Review*.

Gottstein R *et al*. Systematic review of intravenous immunoglobulin in haemolytic disease of the newborn. Arch Dis Child 2003; 88: F6–F10. *Effective treatment*.

Heath PT *et al*. Neonatal meningitis. Arch Dis Child 2003; 88: F173–F178. *Review*.

Leslie A *et al*. Neonatal transfers by advanced neonatal nurse practitioners and paediatric registrars. Arch Dis Child 2003; 88: F509–F512. *Nurses just as good*.

Limanovitz I *et al*. Early physical activity intervention prevents decrease of bone strength in very low birth weight infants. Pediatrics 2003; 112: 15–19. *May decrease the risk of osteopaenia*.

Maayan-Metzger A *et al*. Fever in healthy asymptomatic newborns during the first days of life. Arch Dis Child 2003; 88: F312–F314. *Related primarily to dehydration, breast feeding, caesarean section, and high birth weight*.

Meyer O *et al*. Neonatal cutaneous lupus and congenital heart block: it's not all antibodies. Lancet 2003; 362: 1596–1597. *Editorial. See pp. 1617–1623*.

Macfarlane PI *et al*. Non-viable delivery at 20–23 weeks' gestation: observations and signs of life after birth. Arch Dis Child 2003; 88: F199–F202. *Below 23 week's gestation, none survived, and 94% had died within 4 hours of age*.

McGuire W *et al*. Donor human milk versus formula for preventing necrotising enterocolitis in preterm infants: systematic review. Arch Dis Child 2003; 88: F11–F14. *A significantly reduced relative risk*.

Moss S *et al*. Evaluation of echocardiography on the neonatal unit. Arch Dis Child 2003; 88: F287–F291. *Can be a reliable tool in the hands of neonatologists*.

Nicklin SE *et al*. The light still shines, but not that brightly? The current status of perinatal near infrared spectroscopy. Arch Dis Child 2003; 88: F263–F268. *Review*.

Olsen OE *et al*. Diagnostic value of radiography in cases of perinatal death: a population based study. Arch Dis Child 2003; 88: F521–F524. *Important in 5/542 cases*.

Osborn DA *et al*. Hemodynamic and antecedent risk factors of early and late periventricular/intraventricular hemorrhage in premature infants. Pediatrics 2003; 112: 33–39. *Early and late haemorrhage have different risk factors*.

Parry G *et al*. CRIB II: an update of the clinical risk index for babies' score. Lancet; 361: 1789–1791. *Recalibrated and simplified scoring system*.

Rainer C *et al*. Breast deformity in adolescence as a result of pneumothorax drainage during neonatal intensive care. Pediatrics 2003; 111: 80–86. *Can be avoided by correct technique*.

Saugstad OD *et al*. Resuscitation of newborn infants with 21% or 100% oxygen: follow-up at 18 to 24 months. Pediatrics 2003; 112: 296–300. *Resuscitation with air seems to be safe*.

Schreiber MD *et al.* Inhaled nitric oxide in premature infants with the respiratory distress syndrome. N Engl J Med 2003; 349: 2099–2106. *Decreases the incidence of chronic lung disease and death. See also pp. 2157–2159.*

Stevens JP *et al.* Long term outcome of neonatal meningitis. Arch Dis Child 2003; 88: F179–F184. *Severe neurodisability and milder motor and psychometric impairment.*

Surenthiran SS *et al.* Noise levels within the ear and post-nasal space in neonates in intensive care. Arch Dis Child 2003; 88: F315–F318. *High noise intensities of those receiving CPAP.*

Vento M *et al.* Oxidative stress in asphyxiated term infants resuscitated with 100% oxygen. J Pediatr 2003; 142: 240–246. *Room air may be preferred.*

Welty SE *et al.* Antioxidants and oxidations in bronchopulmonary dysplasia: there are no easy answers. J Pediatr 2003; 143: 697–698. *Editorial. See also pp. 713–719.*

Whitelaw A *et al.* Phase 1 trial of prevention of hydrocephalus after intraventricular hemorrhage in newborn infants by drainage, irrigation, and fibrinolytic therapy. Pediatrics 2003; 111: 759–765. *Shunt surgery mortality and disability rates all showed downward trends.*

Williams O *et al.* Extubation failure due to phrenic nerve injury. Arch Dis Child 2003; 88: F72–F73. *Case report.*

Wood NS *et al.* The EPICure study: growth and associated problems in children born at 25 weeks of gestational age or less. Arch Dis Child 2003; 88: F492–F500. *Poor growth in early childhood is common.*

NEPHROLOGY

Struthers S *et al.* Parental reporting of smelly urine and urinary tract infection. Arch Dis Child 2003; 88: 250–252. *Asking parents about urine smell is unlikely to be of benefit.*

Wheeler D *et al.* Antibiotics and surgery for vesicouretic reflux: a meta-analysis of randomised controlled trials. Arch Dis Child 2003; 88: 688–694. *It is uncertain whether the identification and treatment of children with reflux confers clinically important benefit.*

NEUROLOGY

Ben-Pazi H *et al.* Parkinsonian features after streptococcal pharyngitis. J Pediatr 2003; 143: 267–269. *Case report.*

Colver AF *et al.* The term diplegia should be abandoned. Arch Dis Child 2003; 88: 286–290. *Review.*

Coulthard MG *et al.* A nurse led education and direct access service for the management of urinary tract infections in children: prospective controlled trial. BMJ 2003; 88: 656–659. *Improved the management.*

Coward RJM *et al.* Epidemiology of paediatric renal stone disease in the UK. Arch Dis Child 2003; 88: 962–965. *Underlying metabolic causes are common.*

Eddy AE *et al.* Nephrotic syndrome in childhood. Lancet 2003; 362: 629–639. *Review.*

Hardart MDM *et al.* Spinal muscular atrophy-type 1. Arch Dis Child 2003; 88: 848–850. *Review of management options.*

Hoberman A *et al.* Imaging studies after a first febrile urinary tract infection in young children. N Engl J Med 2003; 348: 195–202. *Ultrasound performed at the time of acute illness is of limited value. See also pp. 251–252.*

McLeod KA *et al.* Syncope in childhood. Arch Dis Child 2003; 88: 350–353. *Review.*

McLeod KA *et al.* Bladder dysfunction in Duchenne muscular dystrophy. Arch Dis Child 2003; 88: 347–349. *46/88 boys interviewed had urinary problems.*

Quionlivan RM *et al.* Central core disease: clinical, pathological, and genetic features. Arch Dis Child 2003; 88: 1051–1055. *Report of 11 cases.*

Shaffer L *et al.* Can mild head injury cause ischaemic stroke? Arch Dis Child 2003; 88: 267–269. *Report of 5 cases.*

EPILEPSY

Appleton RE. Mortality in paediatric epilepsy. Arch Dis Child 2003; 88: 1091–1094. *Review.*

Chang BS *et al.* Epilepsy. N Engl J Med 2003; 349: 1257–1266. *Review.*

Clayton PT *et al.* Neonatal epileptic encephalopathy. Lancet 2003; 361: 1614–1614. *Explains pyridoxal-P pathways.*

Egger J *et al.* Benign sleep myoclonus in infancy mistaken for epilepsy. BMJ 2003; 326: 975–976. *Report of 15 cases.*

Sharma S *et al.* The role of emergent neuroimaging in children with new-onset afebrile seizures. Pediatrics 2003; 111: 1–5. *Clinically significant abnormal neuroimaging occurred with relatively low frequency. See also pp. 194–196.*

OPHTHALMOLOGY

American Academy of Pediatrics. Eye examination in infants, children, and young adults by pediatricians. Pediatrics 2003; 111: 902–907. *Policy statement.*
Gilbert C *et al.* Blindness in children. BMJ 2003; 327: 760–761. *Editorial.*

Rahi JS *et al.* Severe visual impairment and blindness in children in the UK. Lancet 2003; 362: 1359–1365. *Study of 439 cases.*

Sikander SS *et al.* Fear of the dark in children: is stationary night blindness the cause? Arch Dis Child 2003; 326: 211–212. *Two cases of congenital stationary night blindness.*

ORTHOPAEDICS

Brown J *et al.* Efficiency of alternative policy options for screening for developmental dysplasia of the hip in the United Kingdom. Arch Dis Child 2003; 88: 760–766. *Discussion of different strategies.*

Dezateux C *et al.* Performance, treatment pathways, and effects of alternative policy options for screening for developmental dysplasia of the hip in the United Kingdom 2003; 88: 753–759. *Ultrasound based screening strategies the most sensitive and effective.*

Eastwood DM. Neonatal hip screening. Lancet 2003; 361: 595–597. *Review.*

Elbourne D *et al.* Ultrasonography in the diagnosis and management of developmental hip dysplasia (UK Hip Trial): clinical and economic results of a multicentre randomised controlled trial. Lancet 2003; 360: 2009–2017. *Ultrasonography allows abduction splinting rates to be reduced.*

Wharton B *et al.* Rickets. Lancet 2003; 362: 1389–1400. *Review.*

PSYCHIATRY

Afzal N *et al.* Constipation with acquired megarectum in children with autism. Pediatrics 2003; 112: 939–942. *Constipation is a frequent finding in autism.*

Baird G *et al.* Diagnosis of autism. BMJ 2003; 327: 488–493. *Review.*

Burgos-Vargas R *et al.* Juvenile onset spondyloarthropathies: therapeutic aspects. Arch Dis Child 2003; 88: 312–318. *Review.*

Cleary AG *et al.* Intra-articular corticosteroid injections in juvenile idiopathic arthritis. Arch Dis Child 2003; 88: 192–196. *Review.*

Fekkes M *et al.* Bullying behaviour and associations with psychosomatic complaints and depression in victims. J Pediatr 2003; 144: 17–22. *Strong association between being bullied and a wide range of psychosomatic symptoms and depression.*

Gillberg C *et al.* Deficits in attention, motor control, and perception: a brief review. Arch Dis Child 2003; 88: 904–910. *Review.*

Levy SE *et al.* Children with autistic spectrum disorders. I: comparison of placebo and single dose of human synthetic secretin. Arch Dis Child 2003; 88: 731–736. *Not effective. See also pp. 737–739.*

Lingam R *et al.* Prevalence of autism and parentally reported triggers in a north east London population. Arch Dis Child 2003; 88: 666–670. *The prevalence which was apparently rising from 1979 to 1992, reached a plateau from 1992 to 1996.*

Patel MX *et al.* Chronic fatigue syndrome in children: a cross sectional survey. Arch Dis Child 2003; 88: 894–898. *Return to normal health or significant overall improvement was reported by 29/36 subjects.*

Ramanan AV *et al.* Use of methotrexate in juvenile idiopathic arthritis. Arch Dis Child 2003; 88: 197–200. *Review.*

Sowell ER *et al.* Cortical abnormalities in children and adolescents with attention-deficit hyperactivity disorder. Lancet; 362: 1699–1707. *Abnormal morphology was noted in the frontal cortices.*

Volkmar FR *et al.* Autism. Lancet 2003; 362: 1133–1141. *Review.*

Watson KD *et al.* Low back pain in schoolchildren: the role of mechanical and psychosocial factors. Arch Dis Child 2003; 88: 12–17. *Strong associations with emotional problems conduct problems, headaches, abdominal pain, sore throats and daytime tiredness.*

Wedderburn LR *et al.* Autologous haematopoietic stem cell transplantation in juvenile idiopathic arthritis. Arch Dis Child 2003; 88: 201–205. *Review.*

West AF *et al.* Containing anxiety in the management of constipation. Arch Dis Child 2003; 88: 1038–1039. *Review.*

Wilkinson N *et al.* Biologic therapies for juvenile arthritis. Arch Dis Child 2003; 88: 186–191. *Review.*

RESPIRATORY

Amirav I *et al.* Nebuliser hood compared to mask in wheezy infants: aerosol therapy without tears. Arch Dis Child 2003; 88: 719–723. *Hood is as efficient as mask.*

Blackburn C *et al.* Effect of strategies to reduce exposure of infants to environmental tobacco smoke in the home: cross sectional survey. BMJ 2003; 327: 257–260. *Anything less than banning smoking in the home had no effect.*

Brooks LJ *et al.* Enuresis in children with sleep apnea. J Pediatr 2003; 142: 515–518. *High prevalence.*

Csonka P *et al.* Oral prednisolone in the acute management of children age 6 to 35 months with viral respiratory infection-induced lower airway disease: a randomized, placebo-controlled trial. J Pediatr 2003; 143: 725–730. *Reduces disease severity, length of hospital stay, and the duration of symptoms.*

Kirschke DL *et al. Pseudomonas aeruginosa* and *Serratia marcescens* contamination associated with a manufacturing defect in bronchoscopes. N Engl J Med 2003; 348: 214–220. *Bacteria cultured from biopsy ports. See also pp. 221–227.*

Oommen A *et al.* Efficacy of a short course of parent-initiated oral prednisolone for viral wheeze in children aged 1–5 years: randomised controlled trial. Lancet 2003; 362: 1433–1438. *No clear benefit.*

Panditi S *et al.* Perception of exercise induced asthma by children and their parents. Arch Dis Child 2003; 88: 807–811. *Obtain reports of exercise-induced symptoms from children rather than parent.*

Seddon PC *et al.* Respiratory problems in children with neurological impairment. Arch Dis Child 2003; 88: 75–78. *Review.*

Stening W *et al.* Cardiorespiratory stability of premature and term infants carried in infant slings. Pediatrics 2003; 110: 879–883. *Not associated with an increased risk of clinically relevant cardio-respiratory changes.*

van Woensel JBM *et al.* Viral lower respiratory tract infection in infants and young children. BMJ 2003; 327: 36–40. *Review.*

Wainwright C *et al.* A multicenter, randomized, double-blind, controlled trial of nebulized epinephrine in infants with acute bronchiolitis. N Engl J Med; 349: 27–35. *No benefit. See also pp. 82–83.*

ASTHMA

Brand PLP *et al.* Usefulness of monitoring lung function in asthma. Arch Dis Child 2003; 88: 1021–1025. *Review.*

Mantzouranis EC *et al.* Throat clearing – a novel asthma symptom in children. N Engl J Med 2003; 348: 1502–1503. *Throat clearing can be a clinical indicator of asthma.*

Reading R *et al.* Emergency asthma inhalers in school. Arch Dis Child 2003; 88: 384–386. *Review.*

Rachelefsky G *et al.* Treating exacerbations of asthma in children: the role of systemic corticosteroids. Pediatrics 2003; 112: 382–397. *Literature review.*

Sears MR *et al.* A longitudinal, population-based, cohort study of childhood asthma; 2003; 349: 384–386. *The earlier the age at onset, the greater the risk of relapse. See also pp. 1473—1475.*

CYSTIC FIBROSIS

Baumer JH. Evidence based guidelines for the performance of the sweat test for the investigation of cystic fibrosis in the UK. Arch Dis Child 2003; 88: 1126–1127. *Guidelines.*

Byrne NM *et al.* Comparison of lung deposition of colomycin using the Halolite and the Pari LC Plus nebulisers in patients with cystic fibrosis. Arch Dis Child 2003; 88: 715–718. *The recommended doses for the Halolite need to be modified.*

Clark H *et al.* The potential of recombinant surfactant protein D therapy to reduce inflammation in neonatal chronic lung disease, cystic fibrosis, and emphysema. Arch Dis Child 2003; 88: 981–984. *Review.*

Drew J *et al.* Acute renal failure and cystic fibrosis. Arch Dis Child 2003; 88: 646–646. *10 cases of serious gentamycin toxicity.*

Kulich M *et al.* Improved survival among young patients with cystic fibrosis. J Pediatr 2003; 142: 631–636. *Adult patients had little improvement in survival.*

Lenaerts C *et al.* Surveillance for cystic fibrosis-associated hepatobiliary disease: early ultrasound changes and predisposing factors. J Pediatr 2003; 143: 343–350. *Ultrasound is an early marker.*

Narang A *et al.* Oral health and related factors in cystic fibrosis and other chronic respiratory disorders. Arch Dis Child 2003; 88: 702–707. *Enamel defects are more common.*

Nixon GM *et al.* Female sexual health care in cystic fibrosis. Arch Dis Child 2003; 88: 265–266. *Few parents had spoken to their doctor about these issues.*

Ratjen F *et al.* Cystic fibrosis. Lancet 2003; 361: 681–689. *Review.*

Solomon M *et al.* Glucose intolerance in children with cystic fibrosis 2003; 142: 128–132. *16 of 94 (17%) aged under 18 years had impaired glucose tolerance and 4 of 94 (4.3%) had CF-related diabetes without fasting hyperglycemia. See also pp. 97–99.*

van Hoorn JHL *et al.* Vitamin K supplementation in cystic fibrosis. Arch Dis Child 2003; 88: 974–975. *Review.*

SURGERY

Farmer D *et al.* Fetal surgery. Arch Dis Child 2003; 88: 708–711. *Editorial.*

Hilliard TN *et al.* Management of parapneumonic effusion and empyema. Arch Dis Child 2003; 88: 915–917. *Early surgery is associated with a favourable outcome.*

Jaffe A *et al.* Thoracic empyema. Arch Dis Child 2003; 88: 839–841. *Review. See also pp. 842–843.*

Rangecroft L *et al.* Surgical management of ambiguous genitalia. Arch Dis Child 2003; 88: 799–801. *Review.*

Satish B *et al.* Management of thoracic empyema in childhood: does the pleural thickening matter? Arch Dis Child 2003; 88: 918–921. *Decortication is not necessary to prevent long-term problems with pleural thickening.*

Webb NJA *et al.* Renal transplantation. Arch Dis Child 2003; 88: 844–847. *Review.*

Zitsman JL *et al.* Current concepts in minimal access surgery for children. Pediatrics 2003; 111: 1239–1252. *Review.*

THERAPEUTICS

Calvert P *et al.* Restrained rehabilitation: an approach to children and adolescents with unexplained signs and symptoms. Arch Dis Child; 88: 399–402. *Review.*

Davies P *et al.* The efficacy of noncontact oxygen delivery methods. Pediatrics 2002; 110: 964–967. *'Wafting' oxygen is a possible strategy.*

Ducharme FM *et al.* Safety profile of frequent short courses of oral glucocorticoids in acute pediatric asthma: impact on bone metabolism, bone density, and adrenal function. Pediatrics 2003; 111: 376–383. *Not associated with any lasting perturbation in bone metabolism, bone mineralisation, or adrenal function.*

Duke T *et al.* Intravenous fluids for seriously ill children: time to reconsider. Lancet 2003; 362: 1320–1323. *Review.*

Jongerius PH *et al.* A systematic review for evidence of efficacy of anticholinergic drugs to treat drooling. Arch Dis Child 2003; 88: 911–914. *Systematic review.*

Kearns GL *et al.* Developmental pharmacology – drug disposition, action, and therapy in infants and children. N Engl J Med 2003; 349: 81157–1167. *Review.*

Lask B *et al.* Motivating children and adolescents to improve adherence. J Pediatr 2003; 143: 431–433. *Review.*

Lee WM *et al.* Drug-induced hepatotoxicity. N Engl J Med 2003; 349: 474–485. *Review.*

McErlean M *et al.* Midazolam syrup as a premedication to reduce the discomfort associated with pediatric intravenous catheter insertion. J Pediatr 2003; 142: 429–430. *Effectively reduces discomfort.*

Moritz ML *et al.* Prevention of hospital-acquired hyponatremia: a case for using isotonic saline. Pediatrics 2003; 111: 227–230. *Review. See also pp. 424–425.*

Stores G. Medication for sleep-wake disorders. Arch Dis Child 2003; 88: 899–903. *Review.*

TROPICAL MEDICINE see MEDICINE IN THE TROPICS

Index

Note: references relating to the Literature Review chapter are indicated by an * after the page number.